# THE Sugar-Free SOLUTION™

**EASIEST**
Weight Loss Program on Earth

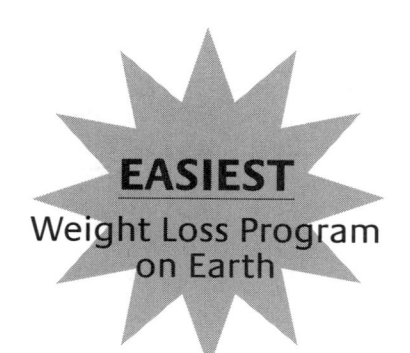

# THE Sugar-Free SOLUTION™

Karen Bentley

www.GETEXTREMERESULTS.com

Suggestions for specific types and amounts of foods are not intended to replace appropriate or necessary medical care. Before starting any weight loss program, always see your physician or health care practitioner, especially if you are pregnant or have specific medical conditions or symptoms. If any suggestions given in The Sugar-Free Solution™ contradict your physician's advice, do not begin the program, and consult your doctor before proceeding.

Copyright 2006 by Karen Bentley

All rights reserved. No part of this book may be reproduced or transmitted in any form or by any means without written permission in writing from the publisher.

ISBN-10: 0-9666-967-4-3
ISBN-13: 978-0-9666967-4-5

Published by
www.GETEXTREMERESULTS.com
A wholly-owned subsidiary of Brook Trout Management, Inc.
P.O. Box 1209
Center Harbor, NH 03226

603.253.4800 Phone
603.253.4801 FAX

E-mail: expert@getextremeresults.com

Front and back cover photo by Ian Raymond
Cover design by The Roberts Group
Interior design by The Roberts Group

Printed in Canada

FOR THE TWO BILLS.
*Because love is the only thing that really matters!*

*. . . true undoing must be kind.*
**A Course in Miracles**

*The important thing is not to strain in any way.*
Bruce Lee
**Striking Thoughts:
Bruce Lee's Wisdom for Daily Living**

# Contents

**SECTION 1: ON YOUR MARK**    **1**

*The Sugar-Free Solution™ promise*    1

Who is this program for?    5

First do no harm    7

How this program is different and better    9

Stopping is a skill that can be learned    11

My story    13

Why sugar makes you fat    21

The case against caloric sweeteners    29

How to identify caloric sweeteners    43

The advantages of abstaining    51

The truth about fats: Maybe it really has been a big fat lie    55

Good fats, bad fats, and in-between fats    67

**SECTION 2: GET SET**    **73**

The four eating strategies that will save you    73

Feeding yourself by yourself for yourself    79

    Grains    80

    Fruits    82

    Vegetables    82

    Proteins    84

    Oils and spreads    87

    Dairy    87

Summary of Sugar-Free Solution™ eating guidelines    89

Is it a healthy program?    91

# THE SUGAR-FREE SOLUTION™

    *Comparison to USDA 2005 Revised Food Pyramid*     95
    *Your scale weight*     97
    *Questions and answers*     99
    *Decisions you make on your own*     103

## SECTION 3: GO     107
    *Get launched like a rocket*     107
    *Now get going*     113
    *GO TOOL #1: Meal planning tips*     115
    *GO TOOL #2: Sample daily menus*     121
    *GO TOOL #3: Recipes*     125
    *GO TOOL #4: Food selection guidelines*     135
    *GO TOOL #5: Start-up shopping list*     139
    *GO TOOL #6: Recommended products, cookbooks and reading list*     151
    *GO TOOL #7: Common FDA food terms*     157

## SECTION 4: STAY IN TOUCH     161
    *Join our monthly mailing list*     161
    *Send your endorsement or tell your story*     163
    *Come to a GETEXTREMERESULTS Boot Camp*     165
    *Share your favorite sugar-free recipes*     167
    *Acknowledgments*     169

# SECTION 1: ON YOUR MARK

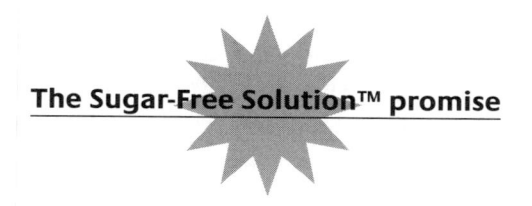

## The Sugar-Free Solution™ promise

Everyone likes to moan and groan about how hard it is to take off weight. In fact, complaining about weight is a national pastime. Just last week, for example, my husband and I had dinner with our good friends Greta and George, affectionately known as the two "G's". Greta is sixty-five-ish and about forty or fifty pounds overweight. Through much of the dinner, Greta complained about how bad she thought she looked and how hard it is for her to lose any weight. "I'm always watching what I eat," says Greta, "but nothing ever happens. It's impossible."

If you're reading this book, it's highly likely that you, like Greta, think taking off weight and keeping it off is "impossible." But I ask you, dear reader, to consider the idea of impossibility more closely. If some villain in the world were holding a gun to the head of one of Greta's beautiful grandchildren and threatened to kill the child if Greta didn't lose weight, do you think Greta might be inspired to find a way to shed the pounds? Or what if some rich and benevolent person offered to give her $10 million for taking off weight and keeping it off? Do you think Greta might be inspired to respond to a generous incentive like that? It doesn't really matter how old Greta is, whether she's pre-menopausal or post-menopausal, whether she's been active or inactive, whether she's never been successful at weight loss in the past, or what gene pool she inherited. The truth is that if Greta really wanted to take off weight, she could and would find a way. Every single one of these seemingly difficult conditions would disappear into nothingness. And our dear and wonderful Greta would finally discover, all on her own, that she was mistaken about the idea of "impossibility."

Wanting something badly enough to do the work to get it is called motivation. Motivation functions just like gasoline in a car. It's the fuel that gets you from point A to point B. It's the fire in your belly, the passionate desire to do something or to be something other than what you are now. Maybe, like Greta, you need an extreme condition to present itself before you feel motivated. These seemingly harsh experiences are actually beneficial because of the hidden motivation factor. Since most of us don't ordinarily have these powerful and compelling life conditions to propel us forward, we have to grow our own motivation. Then we have to nurture it and keep it alive.

Motivation is one of the three critical tools that are needed for life-long success with weight loss and weight management. The other two critical tools are knowledge and process. *The Sugar-Free Solution™ Package for Lifelong Success* includes all three components: motivation, knowledge, and process. This package offers you an extraordinary advantage because it positions you to win—instantly, easily, and with the least amount of effort.

> Weight loss and weight management are not difficult—when you find a solution that's "just right" for you.

- **Motivation.** *My Workbook for Self-Creation* gets you motivated by helping you clarify your goals and by providing you with the opportunity to think about what your life and your body will be like without overeating.

- **Knowledge.** This book, *The Sugar-Free Solution™*, provides you with cutting-edge information about sugar-free eating rationale and guidelines. Everything you need to know about why sugar should be eliminated

## SECTION 1: ON YOUR MARK

from your diet and how to go about doing it is right here, in one convenient spot.

- **Process.** *My Stay-On-Track Success Journal* guides you through a twenty-eight-day process for developing self-discipline, correcting mistakes instead of being undone by them, and appreciating yourself along the way.

In fact, *The Sugar-Free Solution*™ *Package for Lifelong Success* gives you everything you need to launch yourself, like a rocket, and to keep going toward a healthier you.

If, however, you need even more motivation or if you would like to explore the unusual option of approaching weight loss and weight management as a "spiritual warrior," then consider looking into *The Power to Stop*™. *The Power to Stop*™ is an uncompromisingly and radically spiritual program for stopping any unwanted behavior, including overeating. It teaches the little-known practice of "forbearance"—the extraordinary art of holding energy in reserve rather than impulsively expressing it. Even if you have no inner strength whatsoever, you can develop it through forbearance. *The Power to Stop*™ is also a love-based solution, which means that in addition to learning how to stop yourself from doing something you don't really want to do, you are also learning to love yourself—the most important and useful thing you will ever do for yourself and for our world. There is no need for any degree of guilt, fear, shame, or any other self-destructive thoughts you may be holding against yourself. For more information about this amazing and miraculous program, visit www.THEPOWERTOSTOP.com. *The Power to Stop*™ is only available at this Web site and nowhere else.

For now, hold the idea that you are a powerful being and that you can have whatever you want. There are no accidents in the world. You have been searching for an answer, and here it is. The Sugar-Free Solution™ is the key that will open the door that has been locked so long for you. You have just discovered that the idea of "impossibility" is a lie. You are about to discover that the idea of "difficulty" is also a lie. Weight loss and weight management are not difficult—when you find a solution that's "just right" for you. This "just right" solution is now within your grasp.

The key that unlocks the weight loss door is sugar, or, more accurately, it's the absence of sugar. Quite simply, living without sugar and all the sugar relatives such as high fructose corn syrup, white flour, and white rice makes weight loss and weight management natural, intuitive, and easy. If you truly want to act on your desire to lose weight and to stop eating in an out-of-control way, then consider living sugar-free. Just ask this one simple thing of yourself.

Treat it as an experiment and see what happens. Then you will learn from your own irrefutable, firsthand experience that stopping yourself from overeating and losing weight is a surprisingly easy, satisfying, and happy experience. That's right. It's easy. It's satisfying. And it makes you happy. That's the promise! Frankly, what else is there to want but your own satisfaction and happiness?

Not ready to make the decision or still unconvinced? Then at least hold an open mind as you read more about the program. What are you waiting for? Turn the page and get started!

## Who is this program for?

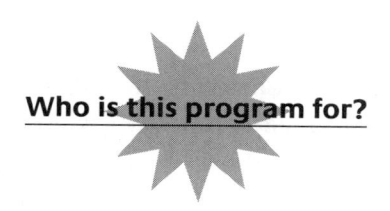

The Sugar-Free Solution™ is specifically designed for three groups of people: those who are desperate about long-term weight loss problems and have not been helped by other, more traditional programs; those who consider themselves out-of-control or binge eaters; and post-menopausal women.

### People with long-term weight issues

People with long-term or lifelong eating or weight issues often mistakenly think that their future is destined to be like their past. This, of course, is not true. It's just another one of those ideas that *seems* true because your vision is limited and you do not yet see or perceive another way of being. There is nothing to fear. Just because you have not yet found the ideal weight loss solution doesn't mean that your problem is harder to solve than anyone else's or that a solution does not exist. Instead of imposing false limits on yourself, why not consider your past as a powerful set-up. It brought you here, to this perfect moment, where your readiness, motivation, and new-found ability connect and make it possible for you to experience a different result.

### Out-of-control eaters

An out-of-control eater is anyone who has a hard time eating just one cookie or one piece of candy or one piece of cake or who finds it difficult to stop himself or herself from overeating for any reason. Out-of-control eaters *know* they're out-of-control eaters. So there's no test to take. If you think this program might be for you, then it's for you.

**Post-menopausal women**

The average age of menopause is fifty. This is when egg production stops, estrogen and progesterone production declines, and there's a general slowdown in the resting metabolic rate. Most women experience a slow, steadily creeping weight gain in the years just before and during this natural but dramatic "change of life." Menopausal weight tends to accumulate in the stomach area and to thicken the waist. Yes, it's a challenge to deal with menopause, but weight gain is not inevitable and/or irreversible.

**The secret to success is easiness and satisfaction**

The secret to your success lies in finding and living an eating program that's super easy to follow and that enables you to experience ongoing daily satisfaction with your food choices. Unless you're a monk, there's nothing to be gained by eating like one and living in constant denial. Nothing! You *must* satisfy yourself with food at every single meal. Satisfaction enables you to endure and to keep going. Contrary to the message in the song made famous by the Rolling Stones, you *can* get satisfaction, and your own personal satisfaction must come to be a priority in your own life.

There is hope. It is real. And it is satisfying.

### First do no harm

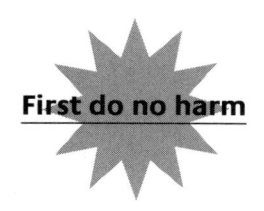

Please first check with your doctor to make sure this program is okay for you if any of the following conditions are present: you have a chronic medical problem of any kind, especially heart disease, diabetes, or cancer; you're pregnant or nursing; you're more than twenty-five pounds overweight.

The Sugar-Free Solution™ is not meant to replace or to supersede the advice of your physician or healthcare practitioner. Do not participate in the program if you have the slightest question about the nutritional adequacy or overall healthiness of the eating guidelines. Discontinue immediately if you experience anything unusual, other than hunger and/or mild gas in the first week or two of the program. Above all else, use your own good judgment, proceed with caution, and do not hurt yourself.

While The Sugar-Free Solution™ is intended to be completely harmless to you or to anyone else who participates in the program, I cannot possibly know what your situation is, how you apply the guidelines, or what's best for you. I am not a doctor, a scientist, or a healthcare expert. Rather, I am a physical educator who is presenting a formula for success that worked for me and that also works for others. My goal is to increase your awareness about the relationship between sugar and weight control and out-of-control eating. I hope that after reading this book you will be inspired to at least try living without caloric sweeteners for a while.

## How this program is different and better

The Sugar-Free Solution™ is based on a simple and easy sugar-free eating strategy. It's easy to understand. It's easy to implement. And it's easy to lose weight. There's no counting calories. No counting fat grams. No counting carbohydrate grams. No counting points. No calculating a glycemic index. No dealing with food exchanges or food combinations. No levels or phases to figure out. All you have to do is identify foods that contain sugar or any sugar relative, plus foods made with white flour and/or white rice, and then make the decision to live without them. All things considered, it's a relatively simple skill to acquire. Everything about this program is simple, straightforward, practical, and easy, except perhaps the idea of abstaining from sugar.

The primary objective of The Sugar-Free Solution™ is to solve the underlying problem of out-of-control eating and overfeeding of self. Yes, of course, you will also lose weight on The Sugar-Free Solution™. Lots of it. And quickly and easily, too! Weight loss is a sure and natural by-product of the program. The primary goal, however, is to learn how to stop yourself from overeating.

> All you have to do is identify foods that contain sugar or any sugar relative, plus foods made with white flour and/or white rice, and then make the decision to live without them.

This "stopping" objective is what makes The Sugar-Free

Solution™ different and better. Other programs are concerned primarily with weight loss. They give you a low calorie approach or a low-fat approach or a low-carb approach or some combination of all three. But what they don't give you is a solution for the underlying problem of overeating. This is why you have not yet experienced permanent success, and this is why The Sugar-Free Solution™ is so bullish about your future.

## Stopping is a skill that can be learned

You are not sick. You are not lazy. You are not psychologically impaired. You are, however, untrained when it comes to feeding yourself, and you lack the basic ability to stop yourself from overeating. And so what you need is a remedial program to acquire the essential "stopping" skill that you lack. If you have been having trouble stopping yourself from overeating, now is finally the time to learn this fundamental life skill!

Stopping is important because when you don't know how to stop yourself, your life doesn't work. Or at least, it doesn't work well. Think, for example, of what happens when you get a new puppy. If you don't teach the puppy to stop peeing in your house or to stop chewing everything in sight or to stop whining, the experience of living with the puppy becomes an unhappy one. You spend much of your time reacting to puppy mistakes and cleaning up after those mistakes. Once the puppy learns to obey a simple "no" command, life with the puppy immediately becomes easier.

The same training principle applies to you. When you learn how to obey your own simple "no" command to stop yourself from binge eating and/or overeating, your life immediately becomes easier. Instead of spending time and energy lamenting your mistakes and making up for them, you prevent mistakes from occurring. Another amazing thing happens, too. You immediately start liking yourself a whole lot more. Why? Because you no longer act or feel like a crazy person; in fact, you are happy. Why? Because, your block to happiness has been removed and regardless of your current scale weight, you are living the way you truly want to live.

Of all the stopping behaviors, overeating is one of the most challenging because you can't just stop eating. You can, however, just stop eating sugar, HFCS, and all the other caloric sweetener relatives. The four stopping strategies for overeating that are presented in The Sugar-Free Solution™ will enable you to stop yourself with skill and grace.

Once you learn how to stop yourself from overeating, you may be inspired to apply your stopping skill to other unwanted behaviors. Any behavior that is unwanted ultimately can be stopped: anger, sadness, alcohol abuse, smoking, taking drugs—you name it. If you would like to learn more about the amazing, miraculous, and life-changing power of stopping, please visit www.THEPOWERTOSTOP.com.

THE POWER TO STOP methodology is radically different from anything else you have ever encountered. The reason it's so different is because it's uncompromisingly spiritual. It directs you *to* love and *away* from fear. Fear-based psychological ideas, group support ideas, or other wildly popular but limiting ideas are not discussed, embraced, or taught. Spirituality is more than lighting candles, chanting mantras, and making a devotional space in your home. It's about recognizing Self as a divine being and learning how to use and rely on your own inherent, fearless, sacred power. THE POWER TO STOP teaches you how to recognize this power, tap into it, and apply it. This hard-to-find stopping information is only available at THE POWER TO STOP web site and nowhere else.

# My story

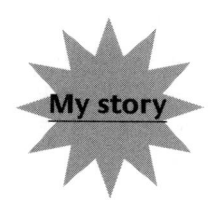

My name is Karen Bentley, and altogether I lost 130 pounds. Not all at once, though. It's a combined total of two separate weight loss experiences of seventy pounds and sixty pounds each. After my first successful seventy-pound weight loss experience, I mistakenly thought I could manage a little sugar in my life. After all, I had been so good for so long. I deserved a little time off. Why shouldn't I reward myself with a dessert now and then? Where's the harm in taking a day off and indulging in a sweet little treat or two? But it turns out that I couldn't manage it at all. In a couple of years, I was almost right back where I had started. And then I had to start all over again with another sixty-pound weight loss.

The most important thing you need to know about me is that I am the real deal. I walk the talk. I will not recommend any practice that I do not personally do for myself. I will not give you information that does not work. I will not make the weight loss process harder than it needs to be. In *The Gospel According to Zen* (Signet, 1970), Robert Sohl says, "If you wish to know the road up the mountain, ask the man who goes back and forth on it." I am the one who walks the weight management mountain. I live on it. I work on it. I play on it. I demonstrate it every single day of my life, and I demonstrate it whether I'm at home, on vacation, on a cruise, in a restaurant, or at a friend's house. I am living proof that a difficult, lifetime weight problem can be solved by an utterly ordinary person all by herself.

There is nothing special about me. We are exactly the same. We probably watch the same kinds of programs on TV, shop in the same kinds of stores, and share the same kinds of family problems that everyone has. My issues with weight and food are exactly the same as your issues with weight and food. I am not a celebrity. I don't have a cast of thousands to do things for me. I don't have a personal trainer. I don't have a team of supportive friends who keep me propped up. I don't lead a perfect life. The world and the people in it didn't somehow magically change so that I would be free of the problems that contributed to my preference for comforting myself with food.

All that changed was me and my desire to be free of my compulsion to eat. I just wanted to be done with it. To tell you the truth, I didn't even really care about what I weighed or what I looked like. I just didn't want to carry on like a crazy person anymore. Once I made up my mind to stop being crazy, none of my past history mattered. All of my past mistakes, and there were many, made no difference whatsoever. Difficult people and inconvenient situations did not interfere with my plans. My current life problems made no difference either. All that mattered was my strong desire, my unwavering decision to hold that desire in the forefront of my mind, and my willingness to try a new formula.

I have steadily held onto my desire and my decision and my formula to this day, and this real-life demonstration of actualized desire is what I have to offer you. You are invited to come and take a closer look at me and to feel my influence in an up-close and personal way at one of my seminars or boot camps. For a schedule, go to www.GETEXTREMERESULTS.com. Or just continue reading the book. It will take you where you want to go.

Everything I do can be easily copied or adapted by others and repeated. I openly and honestly share my knowledge

## SECTION 1: ON YOUR MARK

and experience. Nothing is held back. You get the information and the inspiration to independently guide yourself and to free yourself from out-of-control eating. I believe in what I teach because I live what I teach and it works. I also believe in you. If you don't yet believe in yourself, you can borrow my faith for now, but you won't need it for long.

I have been dealing with weight issues since I was a preteen. Everything I share with you is filtered by my own practical, hard-earned experience of what works and what doesn't. There are several instances when what works for me contradicts the conventional and more popular weight-loss theories of the day—especially concerning the impact of fat and sugar in the diet. For me, fat has turned out to be a great friend, and sugar is the big villain. As you read through this book, I will draw your attention to recommendations that are not aligned with conventional weight loss theory so that you can objectively look at the pros and cons and make an informed decision by yourself for yourself. This, then, is the most useful and relevant part of my story. For those who are interested, here is the rest of it.

> For me, fat has turned out to be a great friend, and sugar is the big villain.

My weight history is identical to yours. I ate when I was happy. I ate when I was sad. I ate when I had PMS. I ate when I didn't have PMS. I ate when I was bored. I ate when I was excited. I ate when I was sick. I ate when I was well. I ate when I was watching TV. I ate when I didn't watch TV. I ate for any reason and for no reason. The first thing I'd do when I walked into my house was to open food cabinets or go to the refrigerator and scrounge around for food. I binged constantly, and I dieted constantly.

When I was younger, I used to diet and binge, diet and binge, and diet and binge some more. When I turned forty, I stopped the dieting part because I was really sick of it, but I kept on binge eating. One day I started seriously overeating, and I just couldn't seem to stop. My longest binge lasted for seven consecutive years. Some days I'd make it to lunch or dinner or even to bedtime without a binge. But I'd inevitably end up eating a whole loaf of bread or a whole bunch of bananas or a whole can of nuts or all of those things together and more. It was not unusual for me to consume five thousand, six thousand, or seven thousand calories a day. My weight quickly jumped to 190 and stayed there for a while. Then after a while it started creeping up again. When it got to 204, I stopped weighing myself. In fact, my total weight loss is just an estimate, because I really don't know for sure how much I weighed at my peaks.

The excess weight made me unhappy, but being crazy around and with food made me even more unhappy. I came to the point where I didn't really care about what I weighed. I just didn't want to be crazy anymore. This was a real turning point for me.

One reason that my binge eating lasted so long is because conventional low-fat diets and low-calorie weight management advice exacerbated my out-of-control eating problem. At the time, I was concerned about nutritional correctness. I wanted to eat *right*. I wanted to live *right*. I wanted to be *right*. Consequently, I bought into the typical low-fat regime of eating lots of grains, pasta, and fat-free foods. It was frustrating because I found it very, very hard to lose weight, even when I was a "diet angel." And even worse, I always felt hungry and unsatisfied living on low-fat food. I'd end up binge eating to get that satisfied and full feeling.

Despite my obvious lack of success, I continued to spend my discretionary weekend time learning how to cook low-fat, nutritionally dense, correct foods. I used to have a whole shelf filled with low-fat and "light" cookbooks. I spent a lot of time reading these books, searching for the perfect recipes, shopping for so-called healthy ingredients, and preparing the most nutritionally appropriate meals. There was only one problem—one big problem. I didn't really like what I cooked, and my family didn't like what I cooked either. Most of the time, it got thrown out or fed to the dogs.

Periodically I also tried an inverse approach to weight management. By that, I mean I totally gave in to my food whims and desires. I would feed myself whatever I wanted whenever I wanted it. If I wanted a Kit Kat bar, no problem. Rush out to a twenty-four-hour convenience store and get three or four of them. I thought I should respect my cravings and respond to them. After all, my cravings were a sacred bodily message. They were telling me something about my innermost need for love and acceptance. I believed that the root cause of my compulsion stemmed from a long-term denial of the foods I most love. The solution, then, was to stop denying myself and to give myself what I wanted when I wanted it.

If I wanted chewy chocolate chunk cookies for dinner, then I should have chewy chocolate chunk cookies for dinner. If I wanted a quart of Ben & Jerry's exotic ice cream for breakfast, then I should have a quart of Ben & Jerry's exotic ice cream for breakfast. This practice was supposed to diffuse and quench my desire. Theoretically, my desire was supposed to gradually decrease in a "natural" way until it completely disappeared or until it operated in a more or less normal range. I tried this approach over and over. I wanted it to work. I wanted it to be true. Yet my cravings never lessened, not even a little. And the craziness never went away. All I got was fatter and more out-of-control and more afraid that Kit Kats and other foods that I loved had some kind of abnormal power over me. Giving in to the desire for food did not work for me.

I experimented with other weight loss methods. One semi-successful approach was to simply pay no attention to food whatsoever and use exercise to control my weight. For several years, I succeeded in masking my weight and binge eating problem through exercise. If I ate too much one day, I could easily counter it by exercising like a banshee the next. This worked well for me when I was younger. The problem is that when exercise is used as an antidote for eating like a pig, it can take up huge amounts of time—as much as one or two hours every day. It's also hard work, and it makes you more susceptible to injuries. After a while, I got tired of all the time and work invested in exercise. I didn't altogether stop exercising, but I definitely exercised less. Unfortunately, I continued to eat more and more. One day I passed over an invisible threshold and exercise stopped working as a weight-management tool. This is how I became uniquely fit and fat. It's also how I discovered that exercise alone couldn't save me from myself.

Eventually, I stumbled into an Overeaters Anonymous meeting and was introduced to the concept of sugar-free eating. While I didn't embrace the twelve-step process or having a sponsor to help me make daily food decisions and to monitor my progress, I was immensely inspired by the sugar-free success stories of members. I also noticed a low-sugar/no-sugar correlation to other best-selling diet books. So I decided to independently try living sugar-free for one month and see how it worked for me. At the end of the month, I was not dying of hunger. I had not binged, not even once. And I had easily lost ten pounds.

I then made the decision to eat in a sugar-free way for the next year. After three months on my own program, I had lost about thirty pounds, and I thought I was done losing weight. So I went out and bought a new wardrobe of expensive size ten clothes. The next month I was surprised to discover the new clothes were too big. I had lost another ten pounds and another dress size. So I went out and bought a new wardrobe of expense size eight clothes. The next month I was surprised to discover the new clothes were once again too big. I had lost another ten pounds and another dress size. So I went out and bought a new wardrobe of expensive size six clothes. Altogether I lost about seventy pounds.

I successfully abstained from sugar for several years until

## SECTION 1: ON YOUR MARK

I experienced a crisis in my personal life and reverted back to my favorite form of comfort: food. Predictably, my weight skyrocketed. After indulging myself for a few years, I once again eventually made the decision to abstain from sugar and white flour. Just as predictably, the sixty pounds I gained came right off again. My weight has finally stabilized.

I lost a grand total of 130 pounds through my two weight loss experiences, and I lost the weight in exactly the same way both times: by getting the sugar and other white stuff out of my food choices. For me, there is absolutely no doubt that living sugar-free is not just the key to weight management but also to my physical well-being. It's the key to eliminating weight as a central issue in my life. It's the key to not being crazy with food. It's the key to feeling good about myself. It's the key to looking good. Maybe it's the key for you, too.

## Why sugar makes you fat

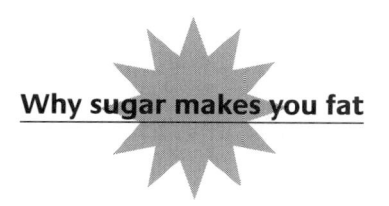

There's a three-way relationship between 1) the highly processed foods and the caloric sweeteners that you eat, 2) the insulin that your body produces to handle or process these substances, and 3) weight gain or obesity. As you will see, it's not so much that caloric sweeteners by themselves make you fat. Rather, it's that the insulin you produce in response to the presence of a high amount of sugar in your bloodstream promotes fat production and storage, which results in weight gain and obesity.

Let's start by identifying a few basic terms.

*Glucose* is the term for blood sugar. Sugar is called glucose after it has been metabolized by the body. Glucose is a primary source of energy, which makes it possible for you to do things such as carrying groceries and climbing up and down stairs. It also enables your brain to do the job of thinking. Altogether there's only about two teaspoons of glucose in your entire bloodstream at any one time. Your body does everything it can to keep your glucose in this tight little range. When your glucose falls below this level, you get dizzy and you just don't feel good. When your glucose gets above this level, you stress your body by making it work harder that it's designed to work. This constant "dis-stress" invites a variety of metabolic disturbances, especially Type 2 diabetes.

*Caloric sweetener* is a broad term that includes sugar, brown sugar, organic sugar, raw sugar, high fructose corn syrup, syrup of any kind, molasses, honey, and most man-made foods that end in "ose." The two most common caloric sweeteners are sugar and high fructose corn syrup, which is also known as HFCS. White sugar is made from sugar beets or sugar cane. Brown sugar is made by adding molasses to white sugar. HFCS is made from cornstarch, which has been treated with acid and enzymes, thereby turning it into fructose. HFCS is not the same as fructose, which is a naturally occurring sugar in fruits.

The term *highly processed* refers to foods that are made with white flour, white rice, or other starchy corn or potato products that have gone through some type of man-made process that involves pulverizing into either a very small or powdery substance and cooking. This includes most (but not all) white breads, most bagels, most cakes, most donuts, most cookies, and most chips.

*Insulin* is an important, natural, and essential hormone or chemical messenger that's generated and released in your pancreas. Its primary job is to regulate or tell your body what to do with excess glucose in your bloodstream. Since your body can only tolerate a small amount of glucose, insulin puts the excess glucose in storage for use later on. Just like airport parking, there are two types of places where glucose is stored: short-term and long-term. Your muscles are the designated short-term storage site for excess glucose, and your fat cells are the designated long-term storage site for excess glucose. The key thing to remember about insulin is that it's the fat-saving hormone. If insulin is present, you are not able to burn fat, because it sends the message to save it.

> The key thing to remember about insulin is that it's the fat-saving hormone.

# SECTION 1: ON YOUR MARK

*Glucagon* is another important, natural, and essential hormone that's generated and released in your pancreas. Glucagon and insulin work as a team to keep your glucose level where it's supposed to be. As you already know, when there's too much glucose, insulin gets it out of the bloodstream and stores it in either the muscles or fat cells. When there's too little glucose, it's glucagon's job to get more into the bloodstream. Where does glucagon get the needed glucose? A little comes from the short-term storage site in your muscles, but mostly it comes from the long-term storage site in your fat cells. The key thing to remember about glucagon is that it's the fat-burning hormone. When glucagon is present, you are not able to save fat, because it sends the message to use it.

> The key thing to remember about glucagon is that it's the fat-burning hormone.

People who are trying to solve a weight or eating problem can help themselves immensely by paying attention to their insulin-glucagon body chemistry and by using food to manipulate this chemistry to be in their favor. Since insulin blocks the capability to mobilize or burn fat, the basic idea is to reduce the amount of insulin that your body produces and still eat in a healthy way. Not only does this savvy personal insulin management enable you to lose weight, it also dramatically reduces your risk of heart disease, diabetes, and high cholesterol. In their book, *Protein Power* (Bantam, 1997), authors Michael R. Eades, MD, and Mary Dan Eades, MD, talk about the impact of insulin on several major diseases: "…obesity, high blood pressure, heart disease, elevated blood fats, and diabetes have a common bond. In truth, these diseases that afflict, disable, and kill so many people in America today aren't diseases at all; they're symptoms of a more basic single disorder: hyperinsulinemia (excess insulin) and insulin resistance" (*Protein Power*, 70).

In addition to generally reducing the amount of insulin your body produces, we are also trying to prevent two conditions known as insulin resistance and insulin spiking. Many people who are overweight or obese have either inherited or created the physiological tendency to overproduce insulin. For some unknown reason, the body starts to require progressively more insulin to process excess glucose out of the bloodstream. This condition is called insulin resistance, because the cells that "sense" or "receive" the insulin stop working properly and require higher doses of insulin to regulate excess glucose. The body, being a good sport, pumps out more and more insulin to try and keep the glucose under control. Excess insulin is a serious metabolic disturbance that stresses every cell and organ in the body. It has been scientifically linked to the increased production of cholesterol; increased production of triglycerides; thickening of artery walls; increased retention of salt and fluid; the inability of the body to absorb minerals like calcium, potassium, and magnesium; and, as we have already discussed, the increased production of fat.

> *In the early 1960s, a research team led by Dr. Anatolio Cruze in a now classic experiment demonstrated the changes wrought by chronically elevated levels of insulin. His team injected insulin into the large arteries in the legs of dogs; each day each dog was injected with insulin in the artery of one leg, and the same size dose of sterile saline in the other. This procedure was followed for almost eight months. Upon examination, the arteries injected with the insulin were found to have a pronounced accumulation of cholesterol and fatty acids, along with a thickening of the inner arterial lining; the opposite arteries, injected with saline, remained normal (Protein Power, 67).*

## SECTION 1: ON YOUR MARK

Some people become so insulin resistant that they can no longer process the glucose in their blood even though they are regularly producing large quantities of insulin. This condition is called Type 2 diabetes. The difference between Type 1 and Type 2 diabetes has to do with the presence or absence of insulin. With Type 1 diabetes, the body does not produce enough insulin, and so, it must be pharmaceutically created and injected into the bloodstream. With Type 2 diabetes, the body produces lots of insulin, but the insulin no longer works to regulate glucose. Type 1 diabetics are not typically overweight because they do not have excess insulin in their bloodstream. Whereas Type 2 diabetics are usually overweight or obese, because they are overproducing insulin and are constantly being barraged with a "save the fat" hormonal message.

There's no shot or pill that you can take to reduce the amount of insulin your body produces. The one and only way to do it is through food. And the type of food that has the biggest impact on insulin production is carbohydrates. The carbohydrate category is a large and confusing one, because there are so many different kinds of foods included in it. Vegetables; fruits and fruit juices; breads, cereals, cakes, cookies, donuts, and crackers; pastas; rice; all caloric sweeteners including white sugar, brown sugar, raw sugar, honey, syrup, and molasses; all caloric drinks; and all alcoholic drinks are carbohydrates. Even some dairy products are predominantly carbohydrates, especially many low-fat type products.

Every single variety of carbohydrate converts to glucose. And, as we already discussed, glucose is absolutely essential for energy, basic life functioning, and optimum health. Since the elimination of carbohydrates is the quickest way to reduce the amount of insulin your body produces, many people are tempted to simply cut them out altogether or to only eat as little of them as possible. This approach works, but it's overkill. You're eliminating more than is necessary to get a result. Life is hard enough. Why make it harder than it needs to be? This is why The Sugar-Free Solution™ is NOT a low-carbohydrate approach. Rather, it focuses on eliminating man-made caloric sweeteners and carefully controlling the intake of other processed carbohydrates. This is enough to ask of yourself. And this is enough to do the weight loss trick.

The second condition to prevent is insulin spiking. When you eat a lot of highly refined foods or foods made with caloric sweeteners, too much glucose gets into your blood too fast. This fast, sharp rise in glucose is called a glucose spike. Your body takes care of the glucose spike with a fast, sharp rise in insulin, which is likewise called an insulin spike. The more glucose you have in your bloodstream, the more insulin your body produces to take care of it. The more insulin you produce, the fatter you get. It's as uncomplicated as that. This high intensity spiking action is what you want to prevent. Naturally occurring sugars that are found in unprocessed fruits and vegetables are easier and less stressful for the body to metabolize and are less likely to result in insulin spikes. This is because the fiber in these foods slows the absorption of glucose.

The other two categories of foods, fats and proteins, usually work as "stabilizers" of glucose. The metabolism of fats and proteins is a slower, multi-step conversion process. When carbohydrates are eaten with fats and proteins, as they usually are in a typical meal, the rate that glucose enters the bloodstream is slowed down and the potency is diluted. This is what is meant by having a "stabilizing" effect.

Several best-selling diet books present conclusive research about the link between insulin production, highly refined carbohydrates, and weight management. They all promote a strategy that restricts carbohydrates (especially highly processed carbohydrates) in one way or another. Some of the more familiar titles include *Dr. Atkin's New Diet Revolution*, *The South Beach Diet*, *The Zone*, *The Carbohydrate Addict's Diet*, *Protein Power*, and all the weight loss/cookbooks by Suzanne Somers.

# SECTION 1: ON YOUR MARK

These books are bestsellers for a reason, and that reason is this: insulin management works!

*The Sugar-Free Solution*™ distinguishes itself from the fine books listed above because it simplifies the weight-loss process by focusing on one strategic and powerful change: the elimination or reduction of caloric sweeteners from the diet. It's also less restrictive than other eating programs. The end result is a super-practical and easy eating program that's easy to understand, easy to implement, and easy to stick to. The simplification process is a great advantage to you, because it strengthens the probability that you will succeed on the program. There's no heavy duty reading to wade through, no counting, no food combining, no special foods, no phases to learn, no levels, no big list of restricted foods to remember. Nothing complicated whatsoever. You get a powerful and easy eating strategy. It's presented to you in understandable, doable terms. And, you get the results you want!

## The case against caloric sweeteners

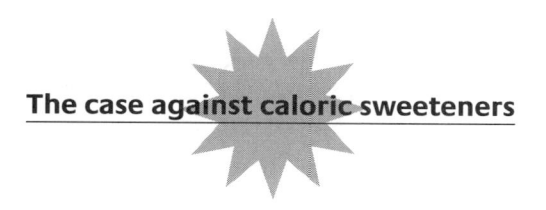

"Sugar is a metabolic poison." —Robert C. Atkins, MD

During his first election campaign, Bill Clinton's campaign strategy revolved around what his new administration would do to fix our national economy, which at the time, was in the tank. Many people were suffering because they didn't have jobs, couldn't pay their monthly mortgage, or didn't have enough money to make ends meet. Yet other campaigners didn't put the same priority on fixing the economy as Clinton did. The importance of the issue wasn't as obvious to them. Clinton kept repeating the same simple "It's the economy, stupid!" message to his strategists and campaigners. The phrase became his moniker, a shorthand way for him to quickly remind his team about the fundamental importance of a healthy and robust economy. The phrase also enabled Clinton to clearly differentiate himself from other campaigners and cut to the biggest problem that most Americans wanted resolved.

**This, dear readers, is my "it's the sugar, stupid!" campaign.** Dietary fat is not your problem. The sugar and the high fructose corn syrup that you eat are the culprits.

Sugar and high fructose corn syrup (HFCS) are the two most common caloric sweeteners that are added to foods in the U.S. Sugar first became widely available and affordable in the United States in the early 1900s with the introduction of Coca-Cola and Hershey's chocolate. Up until then, man-made sugar was more likely to be used as medicine, on special occasions, or as an exclusive and expensive food that was only available to the rich. For the next seventy years, sugar continued to gain in popularity and usage. Then in the 1970s, a new sweetening product, HFCS, also became widely available. HFCS quickly became the preferred sweetener of choice used by many food manufacturers.

Why? It's sweeter than sugar, cheaper to produce, and more soluble. It's also easier to store and easier to ship. HFCS is found in virtually all processed foods including sodas, baked goods, cereals, pasta, spaghetti sauce, ketchup, canned fruits, fruit juices, jams, jellies, so-called health food bars, yogurts, and other dairy products. Go check some of the boxes, jars, and cans in your own pantry. HFCS is probably the dominant sweetener in most of them.

There's no way to directly measure total HFCS use; however, it's estimated that it accounts for at least 50 percent of the caloric sweeteners we consume. Maybe more.

The increased consumption of HFCS in the United States parallels the rapid increase in obesity and Type 2 diabetes in our country over the past twenty years.

Consumption of all man-made caloric sweeteners has been rising consistently for the last decade, increasing by a total of 28 percent. This is a faster rate of acceleration than the rate of growth for the U.S. population, which is growing at a rate of 0.8 percent per year. Americans only comprise 5 percent of the world population, but we consume more than 30 percent of the caloric sweetener universe: a stunning ten million tons annually!

Oh, we are sugar junkies! And most of it comes to us unwittingly—in the form of juices, sodas, and other nonalcoholic drinks. There's an old joke about calories not counting if you drink them rather than eat them. Just one typical soft drink has anywhere from nine to thirteen teaspoons of caloric sweetener.

SECTION 1: ON YOUR MARK

Look at the sugar and HFCS in these common nonalcoholic beverages:

**Coca Cola Classic**
- Carbonated water
- **High fructose corn syrup**
- Caramel color
- Phosphoric acid
- Natural flavors
- Caffeine

**Newman's Own Pink Virgin Lemonade**
- Pure filtered water
- **High fructose corn syrup**
- **Sugar**
- Lemon juice from concentrate
- Lemon pulp
- Grape extract (for color)
- Lemon oil

**Welch's Concord Grape Frozen Concentrated Juice Cocktail**
- Concord grape juice
- **Corn syrup**
- Filtered water
- **Sugar**
- and more...

**Gatorade Lemon-Lime**
- Water
- **Sucrose syrup**
- **Glucose-fructose syrup**
- Citric acid
- Natural lemon and lime flavors

> **Polar Orange Dry—made with 10 percent orange juice**
> Carbonated water
> **High fructose corn syrup**
> Concentrated orange juice
> Citric acid
> Natural orange flavor
>
> **Ocean Spray Cranberry Juice Cocktail**
> Filtered water
> Cranberry juice
> **High fructose corn syrup**
> Ascorbic acid

Here's the bottom line:

1. We are eating more caloric sweeteners than the body is designed to handle and process.

2. HFCS has a stronger, more potent impact than sugar.

3. In addition to making you fat, the presence of excess insulin in your bloodstream leads to food cravings, hunger, and the inability to experience satisfaction from food.

4. Consistently high glucose levels may predispose you to cancers, may exacerbate cancer growth, and may increase the risk of death from cancer.

Let's look at each one of these assertions a little more closely.

**1. We are eating more caloric sweeteners than the body is designed to handle and process.**

Our bodies are not made to process and handle large amounts of caloric sweeteners. As previously mentioned, the body can only tolerate about two teaspoons of glucose, at any one time.

## SECTION 1: ON YOUR MARK

The requirement for such a small amount of glucose in our bloodstream is easily met by eating unprocessed carbohydrates that do not have any caloric sweeteners added to them. Problems related to glucose crop up when we start drinking and eating foods that are loaded with sugar and HFCS. This is why the FDA currently recommends that we limit our intake of caloric sweeteners to ten teaspoons per person per day.

> The FDA currently recommends that we limit our intake of caloric sweeteners to ten teaspoons per person per day.

Depending on the source, estimates about the actual average daily consumption of caloric sweeteners vary from as little as 68 pounds per person per year to as high as 170 pounds per person per year. As you can see from the box below, even the lowest estimated consumption statistic is still double the amount the average person can handle on a daily basis.

|  | Per Person Per Day | Per Person Per Year |
|---|---|---|
| FDA Caloric Sweetener Guidelines | 10 teaspoons | 34 pounds |
| Lowest Average Consumption Estimate | 20 teaspoons | 68 pounds |
| Mid-range Average Consumption Estimate | 44 teaspoons | 149 pounds |
| Highest Average Consumption Estimate | 50 teaspoons | 170 pounds |

At first glance, these average consumption estimates seem high, but if you look at the impact of calorically sweetened drinks, it quickly starts to add up. Four example, just four calorically sweetened drinks per day is the equivalent of 149 pounds of sweetener per year. Children and teenagers are the largest consumers of these beverages. Teenage boys typically drink three or more cans of soda each day, and teenage girls typically drink two or more cans of soda each day. Even more, it's estimated that 10 percent of the teenage population drinks more than five cans a day. And we haven't even started to factor in all the packaged foods that contain sugar and HFCS!

The bad news is that even one can of soda may be too much. Read this and weep:

> *"Data collected from a study of 51,603 nurses in the United States found that women who drank one serving of nondiet soda or fruit punch daily, which was sweetened with either sugar or high fructose corn syrup, gained more weight, an average of 10.3 pounds, than women who drank less than one per month. The study was conducted over four years. In addition, the sugar consumers had an 82 percent increased risk of Type 2 diabetes, since high blood sugar puts a burden on the pancreas to produce insulin."* — www.newstarget.com

**2. HFCS has a stronger, more potent impact than sugar.**

HFCS is not a widely studied substance, and the long-term effects of ingesting large amounts of HFCS are still unknown. For now, we must figure it out on our own and maximize the information available to us. One thing we do know is that HFCS is made from a formula of about 55 percent corn syrup (fructose) and 45 percent sugar (sucrose). The corn syrup is a much more highly concentrated source of sweetener, which roughly equates to about a double dose of sugar. So, for every teaspoon of HFCS you consume, you're getting the equivalent of two teaspoons of sugar. The double-dose effect is stronger, more potent, more stressful, and more difficult for your body to deal with and process.

We also know that the digestive and absorptive processes for glucose and fructose are different. Glucose is metabolized in every cell in the body, whereas fructose is metabolized only in the liver. When too much HFCS is present, the liver malfunctions and cannot adequately process all the HFCS.

## SECTION 1: ON YOUR MARK

Test animals that were fed large amounts of fructose developed fatty deposits and cirrhosis, similar to the liver damage seen in alcoholics. Swelling, atrophy, severe pathologies as well as fatal organ abnormalities were observed in these animals.

The shortcut absorption pathway through the liver has the effect of accelerating the way that your glands and organs function. "Because no cellular action is involved, fructose is absorbed 40 percent faster than glucose," according to Nancy Appleton, PhD, author of *Lick the Sugar Habit* (Avery Publishing Group, 1996, 30). This makes it much more likely that HFCS will convert to fat rather than be used for short-term energy. It also increases the levels of fat in the bloodstream in the form of triglycerides.

The super-fast rate of absorption also may be responsible for interference with utilization of basic vitamins and minerals. Instead of being absorbed, these important substances get excreted in our urine and feces. "In humans, fructose feeding leads to mineral losses," notes Bill Sanda, BS, MBA, of the Weston A. Price Foundation, and author of *Something to Think About*. Studies have shown problems with magnesium, copper, chromium, calcium, and phosphorus. So it's not that we're not consuming enough of these substances, it's more that our body chemistry is so out of balance that we can't use what we consume.

Let's focus, for example, on problems associated with deficiencies associated with calcium, a mineral that everyone is familiar with, and the likely role of HFCS as it relates to the epidemic levels of osteoporosis (porous bones) we are now witnessing. According to the National Osteoporosis Foundation, currently forty-four million women have the disease. Foundation researchers project that fifty-two million women will have the disease by 2010 and that sixty-one million women will have it by 2020. Osteoporosis is a disease of the skeletal system in which bones lose density, become fragile, and break. Insufficient dietary calcium is thought to be a contributing cause. If you ingest large doses of HFCS, you may inadvertently inhibit the use of calcium, no matter how many Tums tablets you consume.

And finally, we also know that some groups of people are more sensitive to high levels of fructose than others. This group includes post-menopausal women, Type 2 diabetics, people who have high blood pressure, people with functional bowel disease, and people who have the tendency to overproduce insulin.

3. **In addition to making you fat, the presence of excess insulin in your bloodstream leads to food cravings, hunger, and the inability to experience satisfaction from food.**

Dr. Seal Harris, one of the early insulin researchers, referred to the condition of excess insulin in the bloodstream as "the hunger disease." He accurately linked the presence of excess insulin to hunger. Insulin blocks the release of the brain chemical, serotonin, which regulates the feeling of fullness. Typically, serotonin is released when insulin levels drop off, after excess glucose has been absorbed into the storage cells. If, however, serotonin is not released, then "false" hunger and food cravings are still experienced even though food has recently been eaten. In fact, Dr. Harris said that "hunger of the most ravenous kind is certainly the outstanding symptom" of this condition.

*False hunger*

False hunger is the experience of wanting more food even though you have just eaten an adequate quantity of food. It's called false hunger, because you can't possibly be hungry due to a lack of food. Instead, you're hungry because your internal chemical messaging system isn't working properly. Think of what happens after you eat an Asian-style dinner made with lots of cornstarch, white rice, and other syrupy or sweet ingredients. Shortly after the meal is digested you feel hungry again—even though you have just eaten a normal or above normal quantity of food. This happens because the excess sugar in your bloodstream called for the production and release of excess insulin, which then blocks the brain chemical serotonin from being released.

*Food cravings*

Food cravings are a variation of false hunger. Out-of-control eaters are always lusting for food, because they always have a nagging, hungry feeling. No matter what you eat or how much you eat, you seem to want more. It is simply not possible to feel satisfied or full when large amounts of insulin are present in the bloodstream. Forever link in your mind the idea that sugar in your mouth results in excess insulin in your blood, which turns you into a craving food maniac.

When you abstain from sugar, HFCS, and from foods that quickly convert to sugar, you are making it possible for your internal physiology to start working for you instead of against you. If your bloodstream has a normal amount of insulin, you respond to food like a normal person. Food has no power over you. You are not a hungry, craving maniac. You will not be prone to eat excessively. You can actually experience the sensation of fullness from a "normal" quantity of food. Imagine that! You can be satisfied. You are not an insatiable, bottomless pit after all. You are normal. This is a joyful discovery.

4. **Consistently high glucose levels may predispose you to cancers, may exacerbate cancer growth, and may increase the risk of death from cancer.**

Last year my sixty-year-old cousin discovered she had breast cancer. While she followed the standard medical protocols of chemotherapy and radiation, she also sought out and followed the latest and greatest nutritional advice as it relates to cancer. My cousin is fortunate to work at a large and highly respected university where nutrition is researched and leading-edge expertise is available. Among other recommendations, she was asked to eliminate all caloric sweeteners and white flour from her diet. The basic operating idea behind this recommendation is that excess sugar in your bloodstream "feeds" the cancer and makes it grow faster. In a report to the FDA Obesity Working Group, the Weston A. Price Foundation states that "Sugar consumption is positively associated with cancer in humans and test animals. Tumors are known to be enormous sugar absorbers" (24).

Cancer is the second leading cause of death; heart disease is the first. It's now estimated that approximately 15 to 20 percent of all cancer deaths can be attributed to overweight and obesity. Here are some recent findings for you to consider regarding the role of sugar, insulin, weight, and cancer:

- Mexican researchers recently conducted a study comprised of about five hundred women who had breast cancer and a control group of more than one thousand women who didn't have breast cancer. They found that the women with the highest intake of sucrose (table sugar) and fructose (fruit sugar) had the highest risk of getting breast cancer but that fat intake was not linked to an increased risk of breast cancer. It's theorized that the link to cancer may have something to do with the increased production of insulin, a highly anabolic hormone, which may also promote the growth of cancer cells. (Source: *Cancer Epidemiology Biomarkers & Prevention*, Issue 13, 2004: 1283–1289)

- French researchers also have been able to definitively link obesity, high insulin and steroid hormone levels, and tissue inflammation with an increased risk of various types of cancers. (Source: *Nature Reviews Cancer*, volume 4:579–591)

# SECTION 1: ON YOUR MARK

- On February 4, 2004, the *Journal of the National Cancer Institute* published the results of a study that concluded a diet with a high dietary glycemic load not only increases the risk of Type 2 diabetes and obesity, it may also lead to colon cancer. In the study, 38,451 women were followed for almost eight years. The women filled out questionnaires about their eating habits. Researchers looked at several dietary characteristics that might link to colon cancer including dietary glycemic load, overall dietary glycemic index, carbohydrate consumption, fiber consumption, nonfiber carbohydrate consumption, as well sucrose and fructose consumption. They found that the women who ate foods with the highest glycemic load were nearly three times more likely to develop colon cancer.

- Another important study was conducted by Dr. Jonathan Samet, chairman of epidemiology of the Bloomberg School of Public Health at Johns Hopkins University. Samet and his colleagues collected and studied data from more than one million Korean men and women over a ten-year period. Participants in the study ranged in age between thirty and ninety-five. Findings showed a relationship between higher levels of fasting glucose and the *incidence and death rates from cancer.* People with fasting glucose levels over 140 mg/dl had a 22 percent higher risk of getting cancer and a 29 percent increased risk of dying from cancer than someone with a normal level of fasting glucose at 90 mg/dl. For pancreatic cancer, the risk of death was almost double. Even in people with fasting glucose levels between 110 and 125 mg/dl, which is not considered diabetic, there was a 13 percent increased risk of cancer (Serena Gordon, *Health Day News,* January 31, 2006; *Journal of the American Medical Association,* January 12, 2005).

- And finally, in her book *Lick The Sugar Habit*, Nancy Appleton, PhD, says that "One way in which cells turn cancerous is through a continually upset body chemistry.... If you continually cause body chemistry imbalance by eating sugar or other abusive foods... you will increase your metabolic rate and produce more free radicals. If a person does not change the abusive lifestyle that wears down his or her body, the sick cells will start winning—in other words, the cancer cells will be able to take over the body. A person's genes do not cause disease—rather, the culprit is an abusive lifestyle that constantly upsets the body chemistry" (*Lick the Sugar Habit*, 78–80).

The link between the fermentation of sugar and cancer was first introduced almost eighty years ago by Otto Warburg, PhD, the German Nobel Prize winner for medicine in 1931. His research concluded that all cells need glucose, but that cancer cells need as much as four or five times more glucose than normal, healthy cells. Warburg further stated that cancer cells are unable to multiply rapidly without it. Here's an excerpt from a lecture that Warburg delivered to the Nobel Laureates on June 30, 1966.

> *"There are prime and secondary causes of diseases. For example, the prime cause of the plague is the plague bacillus, but the secondary causes of the plague are filth, rats, and the fleas that transfer the plague bacillus from rats to man. By the prime cause of a disease, I mean one that is found in every case of the disease.*
>
> *"Cancer, above all other disease, has countless secondary causes. Almost anything can cause cancer. But, even for cancer, there is only one prime cause. The prime cause of cancer is the replacement of the*

## SECTION 1: ON YOUR MARK

> *respiration of oxygen (oxidation of sugar) in normal body cells by fermentation of sugar.*
>
> *"All normal body cells meet their energy needs by respiration of oxygen, whereas cancer cells meet their energy needs in great part by fermentation . . . From the standpoint of the physics and chemistry of life, this difference between normal and cancer cells is so great that one can scarcely picture a greater difference. Oxygen gas, the donor of energy plants and animals, is dethroned in the cancer cells and replaced by the energy yielding reaction of the lowest living forms, namely the fermentation of sugar."*

Ever since the 1950s when Dr. Ancel Keys pioneered the first study linking heart disease to dietary fat, other scientists have been following his lead. Over the past thirty years scientific research has been focused on trying to solidify theories about the link between dietary fat and cancer. The results are a mixed bag. However, emerging research about the link between sugar, insulin, obesity, and cancer is more compelling.

**The last word!**

William Duffy was one of the first American authors to draw the dangers of sugar to our attention. His book, *The Sugar Blues*, which was written in 1975 is still in print and is still a classic reference book on the subject. In it, Duffy talks about Nyoiti Sakurazawa, a famous Japanese expert on preventive medicine and Asian philosophy. Here is what Sakurazawa had to say about sugar and Western medicine's reluctance to understand or embrace the dangers this substance presents.

> *Sakurazawa concluded that Western medicine was many decades late in sounding warnings on the relation between sugar consumption and disease. "Western medicine will one day admit what has*

*been known in the Orient for years . . . Sugar is the greatest evil that modern industrial civilization has visited upon the countries of the Far East and Africa."* *He pleaded with Western nutritionists to make the distinction in the quality of food that they mechanically labeled carbohydrates. He begged them to distinguish between whole, unrefined grains as a source of carbohydrates and the average sources of carbohydrates in the typical American diet: potatoes, white bread, processed grains, and refined table sugar.*

## How to identify caloric sweeteners

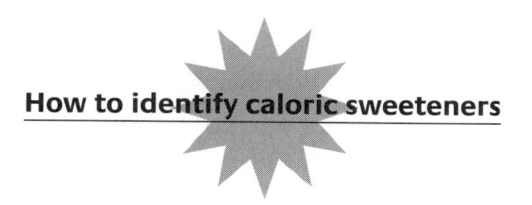

Your new job is to become a caloric sweetener detective. Be on the lookout for any of these ingredients that have been **added** to food products. We are not concerned here about naturally occurring sugars, because all carbohydrate-type foods will have naturally occurring sugars. Instead, **our one and only goal is to identify the caloric sweeteners that food manufacturers have added to foods that come in a container or package.**

**Sugar,** including **raw sugar** and **organic sugar**

**Confectioners sugar,** also known as **powdered sugar** or **icing sugar,** is made from sugar with 3 percent cornstarch.

**Turbinado,** also known as **raw sugar,** is partially processed sugar.

**Brown sugar**

**Sucrose,** also known by the common name of table sugar, is made with one molecule of glucose plus one molecule of fructose.

**High fructose corn syrup,** also known as **HFCS,** is made from cornstarch treated with enzymes, which turns it into corn syrup.

**Modified cornstarch, cornstarch,** and **food starch**

**Syrups** including corn syrup, maple syrup, and rice syrup

**Molasses,** also known as **treacle**

**Honey**

**Fruit juice concentrate**

**Evaporated cane juice**

**Glucose**, also known as **dextrose**

**Fructose**, also known as **fruit sugar**

**Maltose**, also known as **malt sugar**

**Dextrine** or **malodextrin**, which is made by treating starches with heat, enzymes, or acid

As a stand-alone product, sugar is easy to identify. It comes in a bag or a box. It's white or brown. And it's available in the form of powder, chunks, or dots. What's not so obvious is that sugar and other caloric sweeteners have been added to many packaged food products, especially to foods that are supposed to be "good for you."

Forget about all the labels you see on the front of the food package. These will always confuse and mislead you. Even though words like "free," "high," "low," "light," and "reduced" have standardized definitions (which are provided as a tool in the "GO" section of this book), these terms are still confusing for most people. And other words such as "healthy," "pure," and "natural" have not been defined or regulated. Therefore, the words cannot be relied on. Even more, all of these terms are used to sell products and to prey on your belief that fat is the villain in food and that sugar is okay. Many low-fat foods such as cereals, breads, granola bars, and fruity yogurts are the most misleading products of all.

Here are seven perfect examples of how labels mislead us:

1. **Kellogg's Special K.** The Special K brand is supposed to be synonymous with healthy eating and weight loss. The front label says: "Take the Special K Challenge: Lose up to six pounds in two weeks," but it's made with **rice, sugar,** and **high fructose corn syrup.**

SECTION 1: ON YOUR MARK

2. **Nature Valley Healthy Heart Chewy Granola Bars—Honey Nut.** The front label says "helps lower cholesterol, good source of whole grain, good source of fiber," but the very first ingredient is **high maltose corn syrup.** It's also made with **honey, fructose, sugar,** and **high fructose corn syrup.**

3. **Ensure Plus—Strawberries and Cream Shake.** The front labels says "complete balanced nutrition," but the ingredients include **corn syrup, corn malodextrin,** and **sugar.**

4. **Slimfast Optima—Peanut Butter Crunch.** The front label says "40 percent less sugar," but the first two ingredients are **malitol syrup** and **sugar.**

5. **Kraft Cool Whip Lite.** The front label says " South Beach Diet recommended," but the ingredients include **corn syrup, high fructose corn syrup,** and hydrogenated vegetable oil. HFCS and trans fats such as those occurring in hydrogenated vegetable oil are two of the worst things that you can feed yourself! It's a mystery how this food could possibly be recommended by the South Beach Diet.

6. **Wishbone Just2Good Low-fat Italian Dressing.** The front label says "just two grams of fat," but the third ingredient is **high fructose corn syrup.**

7. **Whole Fruit Sorbet—Strawberry.** The front label says "naturally fat free," but the ingredients include **sugar, corn syrup,** and **high fructose corn syrup.**

Instead of relying on words that appear on the front of the product package, go straight to the listing of ingredients. This is where the rubber meets the road. The ingredients list is usually, but not always, displayed right underneath the Nutrition Facts box that is published on most containers. Invariably, the

## THE SUGAR-FREE SOLUTION™

ingredients information is the smallest print. So get out your glasses because everything you need to know to make a food choice decision is right there.

Of course, once you start reading the ingredients on food labels, you'll quickly realize that you have to be much more careful about the packaged foods you buy. Most foods contain a caloric sweetener of some kind. Therefore, your challenge is always the same: to find the foods that are packaged without caloric sweeteners or at least with very little of it.

Here are some more examples of common packaged food products that include caloric sweeteners in the list of ingredients. A wide range of different food manufacturers are presented so that you can see for yourself how common and pervasive it is to add sweeteners to the foods that are typically found in our pantry or refrigerator.

**Breyer's 99% Fat Free Yogurt:**
**Fruit on the Bottom/Red Raspberry**
- Cultured pasteurized Grade A nonfat milk and milk
- Water
- **Sugar**
- Raspberry puree
- Food starch—modified
- **High fructose corn syrup**
- and more . . .

**Starbuck's Lowfat Latte Coffee**
- Skim milk
- **Sugar**
- Cream
- Brewed Starbuck's coffee
- **Corn syrup**
- and more . . .

SECTION 1: ON YOUR MARK

**Hershey's Ice Cream: French Vanilla**
  Cream
  Non-fat milk
  **Corn syrup**
  **Sugar**
  **High fructose corn syrup**
  and more . . .

**Wonder Bread**
  Enriched wheat flour
  Water
  **Sweeteners (high fructose corn syrup or sugar)**

**Skippy Creamy Peanut Butter**
  Roasted peanuts
  **Sugar**
  Partially hydrogenated vegetable oils
  Salt

**Smucker's Seedless Strawberry Jam**
  Strawberries
  **High fructose corn syrup**
  **Corn syrup**
  **Sugar**
  Fruit pectin

**Sun Belt Low Fat Granola Cereal — Cinnamon and Raisins**
  Oats
  Wheat flakes
  **Brown sugar**
  **High fructose corn syrup**
  Raisins
  and more . . .

## THE SUGAR-FREE SOLUTION™

**Hillshire Farm Hot Links**
Pork/beef
Water
**Corn syrup**
and more . . .

**Hunts Stewed Tomatoes**
Tomatoes
Tomato juice
**Sugar**
Salt

**Vermont Maid Syrup**
**High fructose corn syrup**
**Corn syrup**
Water
Natural and artificial maple flavor
and more . . .

**Nestle Coffee-mate Coffee Creamer**
**Corn syrup solids**
Vegetable oil
Sodium Caseinate (a milk derivative)
Dipotassium Phosphate
and more . . .

**Nance's Honey Mustard**
**High fructose corn syrup**
Vinegar
Wheat flour
Honey
**Brown sugar**
and more . . .

## SECTION 1: ON YOUR MARK

You must read the ingredient section of the labels. There's no other way to do it. Please don't be confused by looking at the line that's labeled "sugars" under Total Carbohydrates in the Nutrition Facts section of labels. Remember, that all carbohydrate-type foods have natural sugars, and we are not concerned with this natural sugar content. Instead, we want to know what caloric sweetener has been added and what position it holds on the ingredient list.

Ingredients are listed in order of predominance or what there is most of in the product. So if milk is listed first, then milk predominates. Or said another way, there is more milk in the product than anything else. If sugar is listed second, then after milk there is more sugar in the product than anything else. If high fructose corn syrup is listed third, then high fructose corn syrup is the third most predominant ingredient. Since it's difficult to find foods without sugar and/or high fructose corn syrup in them, a general rule of four can be used to make decisions about foods that contain sugar (or all its relatives). The sugar additive should be at least the fourth ingredient down on the list. If it's in the fourth position or lower, then there's not enough of the substance to worry about, and it should not have an impact on you.

Another problem to be aware of is that products with the same generic name are made with different recipes. Consequently, the additive caloric sweetener content will be different in all of them. The example provided here compares the first four ingredients of three different raisin bran products.

> The sugar additive should be at least the fourth ingredient down on the list. If it's in the fourth position or lower, then there's not enough of the substance to worry about, and it should not have an impact on you.

# THE SUGAR-FREE SOLUTION™

| Kellogg's Raisin Bran | Post Raisin Bran | Grainfield's Raisin Bran |
|---|---|---|
| 1. Wheat bran | Whole grain wheat | Whole wheat |
| 2. Raisins | Raisins | Raisins |
| 3. **Sugar** | Wheat bran | Wheat bran |
| 4. **High fructose corn syrup** | Sugar | Barley malt |

Here's the logic for making a product choice: The Grainfield's product would be the first choice because no sugar or HFCS has been added. Post would be the second choice because sugar is the fourth most important ingredient. And because of the predominant presence of sugar and high fructose corn syrup, the Kellogg's product would not be chosen.

## The advantages of abstaining

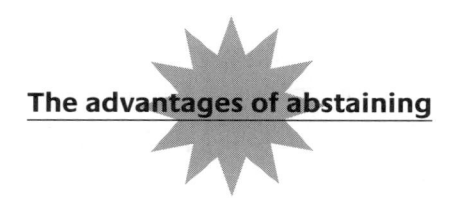

Think of sugar as excitement in your blood, and think of the absence of sugar as the condition of peace. This makes it easier to understand that abstaining from sugar is the choice for being at peace with food. Everyone says they want to be at peace, but this is mostly lip service. Once people figure out that peace is the absence of excitement, the choice for peace is out the window. It comes down to figuring out what you want: excitement or peace? This is the starting place. You can have whatever you want, but you can only have one thing at a time.

Peace and excitement are mutually exclusive. The presence of excitement cancels out the experience of peace and vice versa. The advantage of being at peace with food is that there's no distraction, no drama, no struggle. When you are at peace, you are not at constant war with your physical self. So you have to choose which experience is most important to you. There is no in-between position.

That said, you have four options for implementing the sugar-free approach:

- *Option 1:* Simply cut back on your consumption of calorically sweetened foods and see what happens. This is the most lenient, least structured approach. Many people are able to lose weight just by implementing this one important change.

- *Option 2:* Eat sugar-free six days per week and give yourself a day off. This option provides both structure and leniency, which makes the program doable and livable for everyone. Some people prefer the flexibility that a planned time-off or time-out period provides. It's a compromise approach that lets you "have it both ways."

- *Option 3:* Eat sugar-free seven days a week, but give yourself one meal off whenever you most need it. This option provides more structure than Option 2, but still accommodates a short break from the eating program.

- *Option 4:* Abstain from calorically sweetened substances all the time. Obviously, this is the most structured option. It is the recommended approach for anyone who considers himself or herself to be an out-of-control eater or who has not yet experienced success with a long-term weight problem.

Options 1, 2, and 3 might work for you. They are all a way of gently "leaning into" a sugar-free eating solution, and are better than doing nothing at all. The problem with these options is that you are making an infirm decision, which means that sometimes you say "yes" to foods made with caloric sweeteners and other times you say "no" to them. An infirm decision that waivers back and forth is harder to manage than a firm decision that does not waiver. Even more, a meal off can easily turn into a day off. A day off can easily turn into a weekend off. And a weekend off can easily break your momentum and undo all or some of the work that you've done on yourself. That said, you may be one of those people who can override and manage these obstacles.

Option 4, abstaining, is the recommended choice for two reasons:

1. Abstaining yields the most dramatic and consistent results.

## SECTION 1: ON YOUR MARK

2. It's ultimately easier, faster, and less troublesome than the other options.

Even though it probably doesn't seem like an easy choice right now, abstaining all the time is simpler because you're always making the same "no, I won't eat that" decision. There's nothing to angst about. No pros and cons to deliberate. No need to start over the next day or ten days later or ten months later or ten years later. No wasted energy of any kind. Can you see the elegance and effortlessness of just holding your decision?

Abstaining is also less troublesome than trying to manage the intake of foods made with caloric sweeteners. This is especially true for anyone who considers himself or herself to be an out-of-control eater, because even a small amount of sugar in your bloodstream can dramatically alter your blood chemistry. And your blood chemistry is what determines the messages you receive about cravings, hunger, and fullness.

Even now, if I'm not careful with my food choices, I can still experience uncomfortable feelings of hunger and cravings. Last week, for example, my husband and I ate dinner at the home of some friends. My friends know that I am conscientious and disciplined about eating, but they mistakenly assumed that I wanted to avoid fat. Consequently, they served several low-fat food products that were most likely made with lots of HFCS. I recognized their good intention, and I was grateful to be the recipient of such thoughtfulness and kindness. So I ate what they served. I figured I could dilute and minimize the impact of eating sugary foods by eating lots of veggies and protein at the same time. But the morning after the dinner, I was absolutely starving! It felt like I hadn't eaten for a couple of days. The feelings of intense hunger lasted for two or three hours.

Why deal with hunger and food cravings? It makes your day-to-day life so challenging! By eliminating caloric sweeteners, you can completely change the chemical messages that you receive. Instead of having to override or respond to pesky cravings, you can simply make them disappear. When you "just say no" to caloric sweeteners, you likewise "just say no" to food cravings that would otherwise throw you off track.

You may still have reservations and doubts about the benefits of abstaining. Maybe you think it's too radical or that it's more correction than you need. Maybe you think that moderation is a more appropriate approach. Before holding this prejudgment in your mind, try to at least experiment with the sugar-free food guidelines and see how you feel and how truly easy it is to take off weight. Your own real-life experience will enable you to adjust your perception about the difficulty of abstaining. Then you can make a fact-based decision about how to progress. The perception of abstaining is always a lot worse than the reality of abstaining.

You will come to learn that everything about this eating solution is simple and easy, except the idea that life without sugar is too restrictive, too extreme, asking too much, too this, too that, and on and on. And it's true. Thinking about living without sugar IS hard. But actually living without sugar is not hard at all. This is because sugar is not an essential dietary food. In fact, some experts do not even technically consider sugar to be a food because it's been stripped of every essential nutrient. It is totally optional. Therefore, once the sugar is out of your bloodstream, you do not miss it. You do not crave it. You do not feel unhappy about not having it. You do not lament your life because sugar is not in it. In fact, you start to feel good about life because food no longer has a mysterious power over you. You are free!

> Thinking about living without sugar IS hard. But actually living without sugar is not hard at all.

It takes about a week or two to get the sugar out of your system. You might feel hungry or uncomfortable during this short time period. After that, discomfort either completely disappears or is minimal.

## The truth about fats:
## Maybe it really has been a big fat lie

This excerpt is from the May 2005 *Fit & Firm Prevention Guide* (85):

> *An Argentine is likely to eat thirty pounds more beef each year than an American does—without raising his or her risk of heart disease. How can that be? "The beef in America is grain-fed, but in Argentina the cattle eat only grass, which is natural for a cow," says Alicia Rodriquez, chef and co-owner of Chimichurri, an Argentine steakhouse in New York City. "The beef has about half the calories and a lot less fat and cholesterol." In fact, one independent test found that a four-ounce cut of American beef contained 10.8 g of saturated fat and 328 calories, while the same cut of Argentine beef had 2.5 g of saturated fat and 140 calories.*

American beef is fatter, denser with calories, and higher in cholesterol than Argentinian beef because cows in the United States eat lots of grain and corn, **not because they are fed foods that are rich in fat or dietary cholesterol!** The exact same fattening effect happens to you when you eat a lot of highly processed grains and other foods that have been enhanced with caloric sweeteners. Fat has taken the rap, but how many people do you personally know who overdose on fat consumption?

Do you know anyone who eats an entire stick of butter or a whole pint of sour cream or a whole jar of mayonnaise? How many people do you know who guzzle down vegetable oil? Or who eat a pound of bacon at one sitting? No one. No one does this. But all you have to do is casually look around, and you'll see fat people in Anytown, USA chugging sodas and eating breads, buns, cakes, donuts, cookies, and snack foods that are all made from highly processed grains sweetened with sugar and HFCS.

In July 2002, *The New York Times* published a highly controversial article, "What If It's All Been a Big Fat Lie?" In it, writer Gary Taubes presents a persuasive case that the low-fat theories have dismally failed the test of time. Taubes says, "a small but growing number of minority establishment researchers" are now advocating an alternative, higher-fat weight-loss hypothesis. The basic idea is that a low-fat diet is not necessarily a healthy diet, because it inadvertently leads to obesity and cardiovascular disease, the two conditions a low-fat diet is supposed to prevent. "Public health authorities told us unwittingly, but with the best of intentions, to eat precisely the foods that would make us fat, and we did," writes Taubes. "We ate more fat-free carbohydrates, which in turn, made us hungrier and then heavier."

We have been duped into thinking that just because a product is labeled fat-free or trans-fat free, the product is healthier for us and will promote weight loss. This is because all the marketing hype is on fat, and none of it is on sugar or white flour. The best way to see how we have been fooled is to simply look at the listing of the first five ingredients in three similar cookie products: Oreos (America's favorite cookie), Snackwells (a fat-free product), and Newman-O's (an organic product).

## SECTION 1: ON YOUR MARK

| Nabisco Oreo | Nabisco Snackwells Devil's Food Cookie Cake | Newman-O's Filled Chocolate Cookie |
|---|---|---|
| Sugar | Sugar | Organic unbleached flour |
| Enriched flour | Enriched flour | Organic sugar |
| Partially hydrogenated soy bean oil | Skim milk | Powdered sugar |
| Cocoa | Corn syrup | Organic palm fruit oil |
| High fructose corn syrup | Fructose | Canola oil |
| 53 calories per cookie | 55 calories per cookie | 65 calories per cookie |
| $2.79 for 18 oz. $.16 per ounce | $2.99 for 6.75 oz. $.44 per ounce | $3.79 for 16 oz. $.24 per ounce |

These cookie products differentiate themselves by the type of fat (or the total absence of fat) in the recipe. We can see that the Oreo cookie product is made with partially hydrogenated soy bean oil, a trans fat, which is universally regarded as a "bad" fat. The Snackwell cookie product has no fat whatsoever, and the Newman-O's cookie product uses palm oil, which is a saturated fat, and canola oil, which is a monosaturated fat. Even more, the price of the cookie directly correlates to the absence of fat or to the "goodness" or "badness" of the fats being used. The fat-free Snackwells product is the most expensive at 44 cents per ounce, and the trans-fat Oreo product is the least expensive at 16 cents per ounce.

However, when you look at the predominance of caloric sweeteners and white flour in all of the cookies, you see how they're all much the same. Therefore, despite the fancy labeling and the differences in price and fat content, none of these products are a "healthy" or "good" choice for a sugar-free eating strategy.

That said, most mainstream health organizations and researchers still believe and teach that fat is the culprit in our diets. If you go to a registered dietitian or to a hospital, you will most likely hear the "fat is bad" message and be advised to cut back. After all, there are nine calories per fat gram and only four calories per protein or carbohydrate gram, so it makes logical sense to draw the conclusion that fat through the lips results in fat on the hips. You can tell that most Americans believe in the "fat is bad" message because the average amount of dietary fat has gone from 40 percent of daily calories to 34 percent of daily calories. This is a strong indicator of the national success of the crusade for low fat. Yet something is wrong. Very wrong. Even though Americans are eating less fat, they're getting progressively fatter and sicker with Type 2 diabetes.

Up until 1980, the obesity rate in the U.S. was around 12 to 14 percent of the adult population. However, in 2000, just twenty short years later, the national adult obesity rate has jumped to 30.5 percent or 61.3 million people, with the biggest percentage gain over the eight-year period from 1992 to 2000. According to the National Health and Nutrition Examination Survey (NHANES), **34.7 million American women and 26.6 million American men are obese,** with obesity defined as a body mass index (BMI) of 30 or greater, which roughly equates to thirty pounds of excess weight or more. To calculate your BMI, go to www.nhlbisupport.com/bmi/.

The NHANE survey also shows that **64.5 percent of all adults are overweight,** with overweight being defined as a BMI of greater than 25 but less than 30, which roughly equates to

> If the trend continues, our national obesity rate will jump to 40 percent in just five more years.

twenty to twenty-nine pounds of excess weight. This is nearly two-thirds of our adult population. USA Today projects that if the trend continues, our national obesity rate will jump to 40 percent in just five more years. Humphrey Taylor, the chairman of Louis Harris & Associates, Inc., the famous polling company, says, "Americans are the fattest people on Earth and

## SECTION 1: ON YOUR MARK

are getting fatter every year." The Centers for Disease Control and Prevention (CDC) refers to our national weight problem as an epidemic and predicts that obesity will soon overtake smoking as the number one cause of preventable death.

During the same time period, the prevalence of diabetes has also dramatically increased from 5.8 million adults in 1980 to an estimated 20.8 million people (7 percent of the population) in 2006. Do the math. It's up 358 percent. By the way, did you know that diabetes was the sixth leading cause of death listed on U.S. death certificates in 2002? Or that, in general, diabetics are twice as likely to die from any condition than people who don't have diabetes? **All this risk from a tiny, but powerful hormone that isn't performing the way it should.**

Why is this happening when so many have been so good about cutting the fat out of their diets? It's the low-fat paradox. Even though, as a nation, we're eating less fat, we're still getting fatter. Much, much fatter! In 2004, *PBS Frontline* featured a series of "Diet Wars" interviews with respected researchers and journalists to present us with alternative points of view about why we are so fat and what we can do about it. Gary Taubes was one of the participants, and he explained it this way: "From my fat research, I knew that there were two major changes in the country during that period [the late '70s and the late '80s]. One was, high-fructose corn syrup came in as sort of the primary sweetener in America . . . the other theory was that we started pushing the low-fat diets during this period." Of course, there are other weight-loss research experts with a different explanation. They say that Americans are fatter because we're less active than we were twenty years ago and we're eating more.

Another PBS "Diet Wars" participant, Walter Willet, MD, who is chair of the Nutrition Department at the Harvard School of Public Health and author of *Eat, Drink and Be Healthy*, explains it this way: "The evidence is quite clear that it's perfectly fine to get more than 30 percent of your calories from fat. In fact, it's even better to be getting more than 30 percent of calories from fat, if it's the healthy form of fat. . . . This campaign to reduce fat in the diet has had some pretty disastrous consequences. . . . One of the most unfortunate unintended consequences of the fat-free crusade was the idea that if it wasn't fat, it wouldn't make you fat. I even had colleagues who were telling the public that you can't get fat eating carbohydrates. Actually, farmers have known for thousands of years that you can make animals fat by feeding them grains, as long as you don't let them run around too much, and it turns out that applies to humans.

"The amount of fat had no relationship to risk of coronary heart disease, but the type of fat was extremely important. . . . The evidence we accrued really suggested not only that the type of advice that people were getting was not useful, but it actually could be dangerous, because some people were eliminating the very healthy types of fat that actually reduce heart disease."

One of the challenges that we, as individuals, have to deal with is the fact that the science of nutrition is highly complex and difficult to study. It's also a relatively young science. Results are sometimes presented in a way that seem definitive at the time, but end up being preliminary, incomplete, or inconclusive. And, as in every other science, there is "bad" research: findings that are slanted to favor a predetermined position or that are based on questionable methods and the rush to glory. For example, margarine-type products used to be advocated by health experts as a healthier food choice than butter. But now, we know that the hydrogenated trans fats in margarine are one of the worst, most lethal substances we can eat. As it turns out, butter is a healthier, more intelligent food choice after all. Eggs used to be maligned, but now eggs are good, too. "No research has ever shown that people who eat more eggs have more heart attacks than people who eat few eggs" (*Eat, Drink and Be Healthy*, 64).

Moreover, our government cannot be counted on as a

resource for leading edge scientific information. As Former Secretary of Agriculture Dan Glickman says, the "USDA kind of lags. . . . It does not lead the science. It follows the science. In that sense, the government operates rather conservatively. . . . I think what we've got here is a kind of disconnect between the science that was slow and evolving; the medical community, which frankly didn't show much interest in this issue at all until recent years, and the government, which was trying to provide reasonable information to consumers but always being pressured by the food production side of the picture" (PBS "Diet Wars" interview).

So for now and for the immediate future, the popular opinion of what constitutes "good nutrition" will be a hotly debated, moving target. Given so many contradictions and unknowns, what's the average guy or gal to do? The most practical and wise choice is to keep an open mind, which means that you are open to new ideas as they come along. Here, now, are five ideas about dietary fat for you to reconsider:

**Idea #1: A reduction in dietary fat does not reduce the risk of breast cancer, colon cancer, heart attack, or cardiovascular disease.**

On February 8, 2006, the *Journal of the American Medical Association* reported on the findings of a low-fat diet study conducted on a large group of 48,835 post-menopausal women, ages fifty to seventy-nine, over an eight-year period from 1993 to 2005. Because of the number of people participating in the study, the extended time period over which the study was conducted, and the expense involved, it's been referred to as the "Rolls Royce" of studies. Forty percent of the women received ongoing behavior modification sessions and were asked to reduce their fat intake to 20 percent of total consumption. The other 60 percent of the participants did not receive any behavior modification sessions and were not asked to make any dietary changes. The control group was not able to reduce their mean fat intake to the target goal of 20 percent; however, they were able to reduce it by an average of 8.2 percent, which is a statistically significant difference. Even still, the results were disappointing. The women in the low-fat group did not have a "significant reduction in invasive breast cancer risk," nor did they experience a reduced risk of colon cancer. There was also "no significant effect on the incidence of coronary heart disease or cardiovascular disease." *And even more, the low-fat group did not lose weight.* The diet "focused on reduction in total fat and did not differentiate between the so-called good fats and bad fats," said Dr. Elizabeth Nabel, director of the National Heart, Lung and Blood Institute, the study's sponsor.

**Idea #2: Man-made trans fats are the most dangerous types of fats.**

The "Nurses' Health Study" was published in 1997 and reported the effects of dietary fat in eighty thousand nurses over a fourteen-year period. Once again, it was found that total fat consumption did not correlate to an increased risk of heart attack. So, for example, the women who ate 46 percent fat, which was the highest amount, were not any more likely to suffer a heart attack than the women who ate 29 percent fat, which was the lowest amount. However, women who ate the highest amount of trans fats, had a 53 percent greater chance of heart attack than those who ate less trans fats.

This corresponds to the results of another study, also published in 1997, conducted by the University of North Carolina. The study, which involved about seven hundred women in Europe, showed that post-menopausal women with the highest levels of trans fatty acids were 40 percent more likely to develop breast cancer than participants with low levels of trans fatty acids (*Eat Fat, Lose Weight*, 44).

## SECTION 1: ON YOUR MARK

**Idea #3: Dietary fat doesn't impact weight loss.**

The role of dietary fat on weight loss was studied at a University Hospital in Geneva, Switzerland. Two groups were studied over the same three-month period. Both groups limited their total food intake to 1,200 calories per day. But one group ate foods that had 45 percent dietary fat, and the other group ate foods with 25 percent dietary fat. At the end of the study, both groups lost the same amount of weight.

"In country-to-country studies across Europe, women with the lowest fat intake are the most likely to be obese, while those with the highest fat intake are the least likely. In European men, there is no relation between fat intake and obesity" (*Eat, Drink and Be Healthy*, 57).

A study by the *International Journal of Obesity* compared two groups of people on low-calorie diets over an eighteen-month period. Group #1 ate foods that included 35 percent fat, and Group #2 ate foods that were limited to 20 percent fat. The findings were surprising, because the people in the lower fat group actually gained six pounds, while the people in the higher fat group lost nine pounds. The primary reason for weight gain was that most of the people in the low-fat group were unable to stick to the program.

Michael and Mary Dan Eades, both MDs and the authors of *Protein Power*, explain why dietary fat has no impact: "Of the three basic constituents of food—fat, protein, and carbohydrate—carbohydrate makes the most profound change in insulin, because it makes the most profound change in blood sugar level. Fat doesn't do anything: as far as insulin is concerned, fat doesn't exist. The combination of carbohydrate and protein, especially large amounts of carbohydrate with small amounts of protein, causes the greatest increase in insulin, a

> Fat doesn't do anything: as far as insulin is concerned, fat doesn't exist.

most enlightening fact considering the typical American diet" (*Protein Power*, 36).

**Idea #4: Dietary cholesterol and dietary fat do not lead to high cholesterol in your blood or to heart disease.**

The famous Framingham Heart Study, which began in 1948, and involved six thousand people from the Town of Framingham, Massachusetts, was initiated to better understand the correlating risk factors that lead to heart disease. The researchers found that cigarette smoking, hypertension, and diabetes were all strongly linked to heart disease and that obesity, inactivity, and a Type A personality contributed to the risk. Ultimately, they were unable to prove a connection between eggs, meat, fat, and heart disease.

After forty years, the director of this study, Dr. William Castelli, had to admit:

> *"In Framingham, Massachusetts, the more saturated fat one ate, the more calories one ate, the lower the person's serum cholesterol . . . we found that the people who ate the most cholesterol, ate the most saturated fat, ate the most calories, weighed the least and were the most physically active"* (The Weston A. Price Foundation: The FDA Obesity Working Group Reference Docket Number 2003N-0338, December 12, 2003).

**Idea #5: Dietary fat is absolutely essential for good health.**

Ann Louise Gittleman, "the first lady of nutrition" and author of *Eat Fat, Lose Weight*, explains why we **must** eat fat to be healthy. "Plain and simple, our bodies couldn't function without fats! Perhaps this is why the American Heart Association suggests that we should consume up to 30 percent of our total calories from fat. . . . There really is no other nutrient on Earth that can heal the body from head to toe and keep it healthy from infancy to old age like the essential fats! The big fat lie is that all fat is harmful. The actual truth is that not all fats are created equal. Indeed, they are quite different. There are healing fats, and there are harmful fats. Unfortunately, we have been exposed to misguided and distorted nutritional information that has grouped all fats, from healthy olive and flaxseed oils to the dangerous trans fats in margarine, shortening, and fried foods into the same undesirable category.

"A basic rule is that the body is accustomed to fats that occur in foods naturally. Some naturally occurring fats are more beneficial than others, but, in general, the body can process natural fats much more easily than fats altered by man-made processes" (*Eat Fat, Lose Weight*, McGraw-Hill, 1999, 7–8).

## Good fats, bad fats, and in-between fats

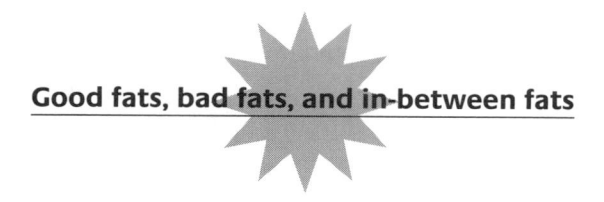

There are four types of dietary fats: saturated fats, polyunsaturated fats, monosaturated fats, and trans fats. All dietary fats are a mixture of triglycerides (which is a chain of carbon atoms with hydrogens attached), but they're chemically differentiated by the number of hydrogen atoms and/or the number of double bonds contained in the chemical structure. Here is a brief summary of the key chemical differences among the four types of fats:

| | |
|---|---|
| **Saturated fats** | Have the maximum number of hydrogen atoms. (The chain is loaded or saturated with all possible hydrogen atoms.) |
| **Polyunsaturated fats** | Lack four or more hydrogen atoms. Have two or more double bonds. |
| **Monosaturated fats** | Lack two hydrogen atoms. Have one double bond. |
| **Trans fats** | A man-made process where hydrogen is added at the double bond site to create a more solid substance. |

**Fat Type #1: Monosaturated Fats = "the good fats"**

Sources of monosaturated fats are olive oil, peanut oil, canola oil, avocados, and most nuts. In countries that border the Mediterranean Sea, people typically eat olive oil and other monosaturated fats frequently and freely, and have been proven to have a lower incidence of heart disease than people in the U.S. Studies involving people and countries on the "Mediterranean Diet" have been a turning point in firmly establishing the healthiness and protection against heart disease that monosaturated fats offer us. With the exception of very low-fat diet fans, which are championed by diet gurus such as Nathan Pritikin and Dean Ornish, there is much agreement in the scientific community that monosaturated fats are not just good for you, they are absolutely essential for optimum health.

**Fat Type #2: Trans Fats = "the bad fats"**

Trans fats are man made by heating polyunsaturated oils to very high temperatures and by using pressure to force hydrogen into the oil, thus artificially "saturating" it. The processing solidifies or hardens the oil, prevents it from going rancid, and makes it easier to ship and store. Trans fat products include margarine, shortening, and manufactured foods made with "partially hydrogenated" or "hydrogenated" ingredients.

> When you abstain from eating highly processed foods that contain white flour and caloric sweeteners, you automatically cut down on your consumption of trans fats.

There is also common agreement in the scientific community that the trans fats are one of the worst, most hazardous substances you can eat. They have been conclusively correlated to increasing LDL (the "lousy" or "lethal" cholesterol), decreasing HDL (the "healthy" or "helpful" cholesterol), and increasing the level of triglycerides in your blood. The man-made hardening process that solidifies these foods also solidifies and hardens your arteries and dramatically increases your risk of heart disease. There is also a study that links high levels of trans fatty acids in the blood to breast cancer.

Luckily for you, when you abstain from eating highly processed foods that contain white flour and caloric sweeteners, you automatically cut way down on your consumption of trans fats. **Trans fats are the only type of fats that The Sugar-Free Solution™ specifically recommends you avoid.** Beginning in 2006, food manufacturers are supposed to label products that contain trans fats. However, you can always double-check by looking for the words "partially hydrogenated," "hydrogenated," or "vegetable shortening" on the ingredient list. Be aware that many foods that are made with powdered milk contain these substances, including gravies and sauces that come in those little paper packets.

**Fat Type #3: Polyunsaturated Fats = "an in-between fat"**

Polyunsaturated fats are found in corn oil, soybean oil, sesame oil, seeds, whole grains, and fatty fish such as salmon and tuna. They're important because they contain linoleic acid, an essential nutrient. That makes polyunsaturated fats "good fats." But there's a catch. When polyunsaturated oils are subjected to high heats, they're converted to trans fats. So, for example, if you're frying foods in a polyunsaturated oil, the oil will be converted into a trans fat during the cooking process. This is what makes fried foods that you get in fast-food restaurants so objectionable. And this is what gives polyunsaturated fats that "in between" sometimes good, other times not-so-good billing.

**Fat Type #4: Saturated Fats = "another in-between type fat"**

Saturated fats are found in animal meats and dairy products as well as in palm oil and coconut oil. When it comes to saturated fats, there are two opposing camps of information. Some researchers say they're okay—at least in moderation—and others say that saturated fats are not okay. Those who believe saturated fat is okay tell us that naturally occurring saturated fats are needed to protect organs, that the body can break down and handle these substances if they're eaten in moderation or in roughly equal proportion to monosaturated fats, and that saturated fats have no impact on insulin production. Those who are not fans of saturated fat maintain that while the case is clearly not as strong as with trans fats, there is still some scientific evidence that links saturated fats to the risk of heart disease.

The choice to eat or not to eat saturated fats is a decision you will make on your own, dear reader. I personally eat saturated fats every day of my life, including fatty meats, cream, butter, and cheeses. In fact, one of the foods that I most look forward to is my own recipe for homemade, sugar-free ice cream, made with a half cup of heavy cream, which I eat three or four nights a week. I have found no impact on my weight or blood chemistry or general feelings of well-being from eating these foods. That said, the decision to eat saturated fat or to refrain from eating saturated fat is one that you make for yourself. You can easily incorporate less saturated fat food choices into the program and still be successful.

**Cholesterol**

In the olden days, twenty or thirty years ago, it was thought that foods rich in dietary cholesterol had the biggest influence in generating high levels of serum cholesterol, which is the kind of cholesterol that floats around in your blood. This is why eggs, red meat, and other high-cholesterol foods were supposed to be avoided. Now, it's generally agreed that dietary cholesterol only accounts for about 20 percent of serum cholesterol. The other 80 percent is generated in the liver, whether or not you eat foods with a lot of dietary cholesterol in them. So what substance or substances does the liver use to generate serum cholesterol? Well, that would be glucose and fatty acids. High levels of insulin also continuously stimulate the production of cholesterol, whereas glucagon slows down the production of cholesterol. The reason that a sugar-free diet has such a positive impact on your serum cholesterol is because you are pumping out less insulin and you are putting less glucose and HCFS into your liver. Therefore, the liver automatically produces less cholesterol.

## SECTION 1: ON YOUR MARK

Cholesterol is another one of those naturally occurring, important substances that's gotten a dirty name. Ninety percent of the cholesterol in your body is located in the cells where it performs essential functions such as manufacturing adrenal hormones and sex hormones. Cholesterol also helps to manufacture bile acids that are used in the digestion of fat. In fact, even the dry weight of the human brain is made up of about two-thirds cholesterol.

The other 10 percent of the cholesterol in your body is located in your bloodstream. Problems crop up in the way that the cholesterol gets transported by lipoproteins to different parts of your body. LDL, or low-density lipoproteins, take the cholesterol to blood vessels, where it gets deposited and does all that nasty clogging. HDL, or high-density lipoproteins, take the cholesterol to the liver, where it gets processed out of the body. This is why LDL is referred to as the "lousy" or "lethal" cholesterol and HDL is referred to as the "helpful" or "healthy" cholesterol.

## SECTION 2: GET SET

## The four eating strategies that will save you

The Sugar-Free Solution™ gives you four practical, powerful eating strategies for taking off weight and keeping it off:

1. **Abstain from caloric sweeteners.** This is the most important strategy. If you only do this one thing for yourself, then you have made a great healthy stride in the right direction.

2. **Eat for satisfaction.**

3. **Prevent hunger.**

4. **Eat a "just right" volume of foods.**

Successful weight loss and permanent weight management is achieved by picking a strategy or a set of strategies that work for you and that you can stick with in a consistent way. Consistency is ultimately the key. As you already know, there are many weight-loss strategies floating around. The secret is to find the one that you can live with day in and day out for a long time, perhaps the rest of your life. What I observe is that most people who want to lose weight aren't consistent about sticking to their preferred strategy. Therefore, it doesn't work. Or, it doesn't work for long.

Let's go back to my friends, the fabulous two G's. The gorgeous Greta, who is always complaining about her weight, mostly follows a low-fat strategy. This is what I see when we go out to dinner together. As soon as the basket of bread appears after we sit down at the table, Greta helps herself to one or two slices of it. If a low-fat type spread is available, she uses it. If not, she uses butter. Usually, she orders wine, but sometimes she has a cosmopolitan instead. If the group is interested in sharing an appetizer, she eats a small portion of whatever is ordered. She typically orders a salad and selects a low-fat dressing if it's offered. If not, then she'll have whatever suits her fancy. Her choice for a main course is almost always a piece of fish or sometimes a piece of chicken, prepared in any way featured by the restaurant. Greta likes to brag about the fact that she rarely eats red meat of any kind. Her main course is typically accompanied by two sides: a starchy type food such as potato or pasta and another vegetable. Then she finishes the evening meal by sharing a dessert with her husband, George.

There is nothing bad or wrong in eating this way, dear reader, and I am in no way judging the lovely Greta, whom I adore. All I am suggesting is that Greta does not eat in a 100 percent strategic way. Her low-fat approach is implemented some of the time, when it's convenient, but not all of the time. Mostly, Greta makes the low-fat food choices that are the least objectionable to her, and ignores the rest. When you finally decide upon a strategy, no matter what it is, you need to be dedicated to that strategy. Otherwise, the same thing will happen to you that happens to Greta: nothing.

Now let's look at each of the four strategies more closely.

### 1. Abstaining from caloric sweeteners

As much as possible, abstain from caloric sweeteners of all kinds. Since caloric sweeteners are in so many foods, it will not always be practical to abstain a full 100 percent. So the question to ask yourself is this: how close to 100 percent is close enough? The recommendation is to shoot for a general target of about 98 percent. This precludes the temptation to indulge yourself, but also allows for the little bit of leeway that's needed for living in our highly processed food world.

**2. Eating for satisfaction**

It's important to experience fullness and enjoyment from the foods that you choose to eat. When you don't experience fullness, you're always on the prowl for something more or something else to eat. Likewise, when you don't enjoy the foods that you eat, you end up counting the days until you can start eating something that you really want. Ultimately, any food program that deprives you of fullness and enjoyment is not sustainable. You can do it for a little while, but not for long. Many people tend to discount the intrinsic value of their own happiness with food. It's as if their happiness doesn't matter. But it does.

The secret of experiencing fullness and satisfaction is to prepare and cook foods with real, naturally occurring fats. The Sugar-Free Solution™ asks you to strategically and intentionally include these delicious and filling fats in your diet to enhance flavors and to curb your appetite. This means that you will be cooking and preparing foods with real oils, spreads, and dairy products that are not man-made, and you will be eating foods that you like. If you are eating foods that are "good for you," but that you don't like, you will not be able to endure for long.

Fats have no impact on the production and secretion of insulin. Therefore, on this eating program, fat is your friend. It suppresses your appetite. It satisfies and makes food taste flavorful. Eating fat is essential for your success at long-term weight loss.

**3. Preventing hunger**

When people finally get serious about taking off weight, they typically resort to the one sure strategy that always works: cutting back on food intake, cutting way back. For most people, this means no fats, no sugars, no volume. Maybe they'll have a small fat-free yogurt for breakfast and a piece of fruit for lunch and a piece of fish with some veggies for dinner. After a month or so, they're really pleased because a lot of weight has dropped off. And again, I am making no judgment about the goodness or badness of taking weight off in this way. God knows, I've done it myself enough times. The problem is that eating in such a minimalist, Spartan way is not comfortable or sustainable. All you can stand is one or two months at the most. The recommendation to eat more and to eat more often seems to fly in the face of the inclination to cut out as much food as you can bear to cut out, yet this is what you are asked to do.

One of the biggest reasons for overfeeding yourself is hunger. If you allow yourself to experience hunger, especially the deep hunger that comes from starving yourself, you ultimately will overcorrect by overeating or binge eating. Therefore, it's strategically important and useful to preempt deep hunger from occurring. You prevent it by eating three moderate "just right" meals and two or three small snacks each day. It's especially important to curb your evening appetite with an afternoon snack that's rich in protein and/or fat.

This strategy of feeding yourself five or six times a day not only makes it possible for you to lose weight without experiencing hunger, but it also serves you in another way by leveling out your glucose production. You prevent those big spikes from overeating or big lows from undereating.

### 4. Eating a "just right" volume of everything else

Advice to eat when hungry and stop when full sounds reasonable, but it doesn't work. People who overfeed themselves don't get accurate or reliable hunger messages. This is why they need concrete, livable, practical boundaries. Like the baby bear in the childhood fairy tale, we are in search of a way of eating that's "just right." Not too much. Not too little. Not too hard. Not too soft. Not too restrictive. Not too free. We are looking for that hard-to-find middle of the road place of perfect balance.

## SECTION 2: GET SET

The Sugar-Free Solution™ program asks you to eat about four pounds of food every day. This is a "just right" volume for making sure that you're not hungry, "just right" for making sure that your nutritional needs are met, and "just right" for taking off weight and keeping it off.

## Feeding yourself by yourself for yourself

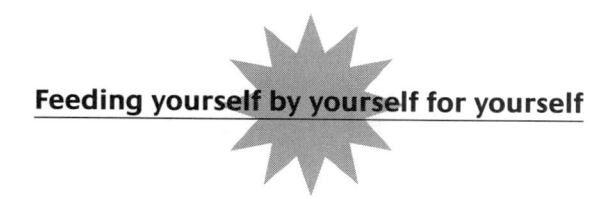

We ask a lot from food. We want food to sustain the precious life force that we have been given. We want food to give us abundant energy so that we can do the things we want to do. We want food to help us resist and prevent disease. We want food to please, comfort, and satisfy. And, of course, we want all this to come about in a way that enables weight loss and weight management.

The food program eating guidelines in this book enable you to meet all of these objectives. They are provided in terms of overall volume, frequency of eating periods, and maximum recommended quantities by type of food. Remember, dear reader, these are guidelines—not rigid rules.

**Volume**

In terms of volume, you will be eating about four pounds of food each day, broken down as follows:

- An abundance of nonstarchy vegetables
- A carefully controlled amount of fruits, grains, starches, and dairy
- An above-average amount of protein
- Oils and spreads for flavor and satisfaction
- No caloric sweets

Before you get started, **buy yourself an inexpensive food scale.** Nobody knows what four ounces of meat look like or what eight ounces of veggies look like. Nobody. Don't trust yourself to "wing it" without a scale. Even I can still fool myself into guessing that four ounces of meat is just two ounces. You need to measure your at-home meals until you gain an understanding of what the quantities look like. This will take at least a month, maybe longer.

**Frequency**

In terms of frequency, you will be eating three meals a day and two or three snacks each day—nothing else in between. Here's a recommended schedule.

| | | |
|---|---|---|
| Early Morning | Meal #1 | Breakfast |
| Mid-morning | Snack #1 | Optional (if needed) |
| Midday | Meal #2 | Lunch |
| Late afternoon | Snack #1 or #2 | High protein or fat snack to curb your evening appetite |
| Early evening | Meal # 3 | Dinner |
| Later | Snack #2 or #3 | Dessert |

**Types of food**

Maximum daily targets for quantities of foods are organized by large category types including grains, fruits, veggies, proteins, dairy, and oils/spreads.

**1. Grains (a type of carbohydrate)**

*Maximum daily target: 2 ounces per day*

Typical sources of grains are cereals, breads, muffins, pizza dough, crackers, pastas, and rices. A grain is a refined or processed carbohydrate. Wheat, for example, might get processed and bleached into flour. Corn might get processed into corn meal. The word "processed" means that some mechanized procedure has been done to it, and the food is not being consumed in a whole or natural state. Processing always removes nutritional value from the food. Therefore, the less the food is processed, the better it is for you—both from a nutritional standpoint and from an insulin management standpoint. This is because processing concentrates the energy contained in the food, which then quickly and easily converts the food into glucose. This, in turn, can cause a sharp rise in your insulin production. Eating a piece or two of white bread might seem harmless enough, but it has the same metabolic impact as eating a piece of cake.

> Notice that grains are not to be eliminated. You must eat grains to be healthy, but not a lot of them.

Since grains have a big potential to impact your insulin production, you have to be careful about what grains you choose to eat and how much of them you choose to eat. Notice that grains are not to be eliminated. You must eat grains to be healthy, but not a lot of them. If you're picking grain products off the grocery shelf, choose products that are the least processed. Look for foods that are labeled 100 percent whole, such as 100 percent whole wheat. Another trick is to check the nutrition label and find foods that contain three or more grams of fiber per serving. The fiber count is another indicator of the wholeness of the food. Pick brown rice instead of white rice. Or consider making your own baked products and doughs from less processed grain sources or from alternative sources such as soy or blanched almond flour.

### 2. Fruits (a type of carbohydrate)

*Maximum daily target: 8 ounces per day (1 cup)*

Fruits have a high concentration of natural sugar; therefore, you also have to be careful about how many fruits you eat.

Again, notice that fruits are not to be eliminated. Limit your fruit consumption to one eight-ounce serving most days and two servings once in a while. Since bananas and most dried fruits are high in starch and are quickly converted to glucose, these are fruits that you can have once in a while, on a special occasion.

### 3. Vegetables (a type of carbohydrate)

*Maximum daily target of nonstarchy vegetables: 32 ounces per day (4 cups). This includes approximately 16 ounces (2 cups) of starchy vegetables per <u>week</u>.*

Mom was right after all. Eat your veggies and lots of them. Vegetables are your primary source of quick energy. They're also delicious, nutrient dense, and fiber rich. The more fiber you eat, the slower you digest your food. The slower you digest your food, the more slowly it turns into glucose in your bloodstream. This has a positive impact on your insulin management. Diets that are high in veggies and other unprocessed carbohydrates can also lower your triglyceride levels and your total cholesterol, including LDL.

Purchase your vegetables in any way that is convenient for you: fresh, frozen, canned, or in a jar. The only consideration is to eat a combination of both raw and cooked veggies, because heat makes certain nutrients contained in plants easier to absorb. Cooking also makes many veggies taste better, which is important.

Vegetables come in two varieties: those that are high in starch and those that aren't. Corn and root vegetables have a higher starch/sugar content than vegetables grown above the ground. This means that you have to be more discerning with your root vegetable choices. With the exception of corn, veggies that are grown above the ground can be eaten in abundance. In the past, good nutrition was defined by eating a starch and a nonstarch type veggie at lunch and dinner. This is no longer the case for you.

Starchy type foods have the potential to produce an increase in glucose in the blood. However, the increase is moderated by the presence of fiber and also because the source of sugar is not so highly concentrated as with foods that have been processed. Also, when these starchy foods are combined in a meal with other types of foods, the impact on glucose is further diluted. This makes formulating a guideline for exactly how much starch is "right" a little tricky. As a starting point, it's recommended that you limit your intake of starchy vegetables to two cups or sixteen ounces <u>per week</u>. This gives you latitude to use these types of vegetables for cooking and/or an occasional side veggie serving. If you want a serving of potatoes once in a while, have one—just not too often. Try to remember that starches are used to fatten cows before they go to slaughter. A lot of starch will have the same effect on you. Again, it's not that starches must be completely eliminated from your diet. It's more that you need to become discerning and careful with them.

Do this for a month and see how it works for you. Then you can make fine-tuned adjustments based on your actual experience. Here's a general guideline for the thirty-two-ounce (two-pound) veggie target:

| | | |
|---|---|---|
| Breakfast: | 4 ounces of cooked veggies | |
| Lunch: | 4 ounces of cooked veggies | |
| | 8 ounces of raw veggies (salad) | |
| Dinner: | 8 ounces of cooked veggies | |
| | 8 ounces of raw veggies (salad) | |
| **TOTAL:** | **32 ounces** | |

Thirty-two ounces is a lot of vegetables, and it will be almost impossible for you to experience hunger with this kind of volume. However, there's one small downside of which to be aware. Did you know that eating lots of veggies can give you gas? When you eat two pounds of vegetables every day, you are eating a lot of fiber. Fiber is good for you, because it aids digestion, slows down the rate of absorption of glucose into your bloodstream, and makes you feel full. But high-fiber diets have been known to produce a lot of intestinal gas. This happens because fiber is not digested. As a result, the undigested food creates little air pockets in the large intestine where gas is produced. The gas shouldn't bother you unless it gets trapped. Also, over time, your body adjusts to the increase in fiber intake and, eventually, produces less gas.

### 4. Proteins: Meats/Chicken/Fish/Eggs/Nuts/Seeds/Hard Cheese

The daily protein budget varies from 12 ounces per day to 16 ounces per day based on your gender and your target weight.

*Women's maximum daily protein budget: 14 ounces (or 1 ounce of protein for each 10-pound increment of your target weight—see examples on the next page)*

*Men's maximum daily protein budget: 16 ounces (or 1 ounce of protein for each 10-pound increment of your target weight—see examples on the next page)*

| Examples: | | |
|---|---|---|
| Target weight of 120 | = | 12 ounces of protein |
| Target weight of 135 | = | 13.5 ounces of protein |
| Target weight of 150 | = | 15 ounces of protein for men |
| Target weight of 150 | = | 14 ounces of protein for women |
| Target weight of 175 | = | 16 ounces of protein for men |
| Target weight of 175 | = | 14 ounces of protein for women |
| Target weight of 200 | = | 16 ounces of protein for men |
| Target weight of 200 | = | 14 ounces of protein for women |

Each of your three daily meals should contain some high-quality protein. Protein generates the release of glucagon, which, as you may recall, is the hormone that gives the message to retrieve and use your body fat rather than to store it. It also stabilizes your glucose levels and helps to prevent spiking. Finally, protein is needed to provide the nine essential amino acids that enable your body to repair itself, fight disease, and maintain your muscles or lean body tissue.

In short, protein is "food" for your muscles. Muscles make you look sleeker and smaller than fat. Muscles make you stronger and more able to do the things you want to do in life. Muscles are metabolically active, which means that they burn energy rather than store it like fat. Muscles prevent your bones and joints from injury and dysfunction. And perhaps most importantly, your muscles play a major role in how much glucagon is released.

Protein has little effect on increasing the glucose in your blood. That said, the "right" amount of daily protein is another one of those highly controversial and hotly debated topics. The USDA Pyramid guideline displayed on page 89 recommends up to a maximum of 6.5 ounces of protein per day for young males. Other than Hollywood starlets, most American adults cruise right by the 6.5-ounce target in one meal. Then on the other end of the spectrum is the Atkins diet with an unlimited protein budget. In between, there are complicated formulas for calculating your ideal protein consumption using grams (a unit of measure that most American adults are not familiar with) plus your current lean body mass and your current level of regular exercise or activity.

The Sugar-Free Solution™ provides a quick and simple protein guideline, which is calculated using one ounce of protein for each ten pounds in your target weight, up to a maximum of fourteen ounces a day for women and sixteen ounces a day for men. Even though The Sugar-Free Solution™ protein budget is larger than most other weight-loss programs, it is still less than you are probably used to eating. Because of this, please be sure to weigh your protein portions. Otherwise, you will be playing a little game where fooling yourself is okay.

Here's an example of how a protein target of thirteen ounces per day and a protein target of sixteen ounces might be portioned throughout one day:

| Example #1: | Daily protein target of 13 ounces |
|---|---|
| Breakfast: | 2 ounces |
| Lunch: | 4 ounces |
| Snack: | 2 ounces |
| Dinner: | 5 ounces |
| **Total:** | **13 ounces** |
| **Example #2:** | **Daily protein target of 16 ounces** |
| Breakfast: | 2 ounces |
| Lunch: | 6 ounces |
| Snack: | 2 ounces |
| Dinner: | 6 ounces |
| **Total:** | **16 ounces** |

5. **Oils and spreads (types of fats)**

*Daily target: As needed for cooking, flavor, and satisfaction*

It's not necessary to measure your daily intake of fat, because fat has no impact on insulin production. However, there's nothing useful to be gained by overdoing it with fats. Use what you need, and leave it at that. You can cook and flavor foods with oils, butter, and other spreads. Remember that the only "bad" fats in The Sugar-Free Solution™ are man-made trans fats, which includes margarine, shortening, and "partially hydrogenated" or "hydrogenated" food products. So be sure to get those trans fat products out of your refrigerator. Also recall that polyunsaturated oils have the potential to convert to trans fats when they're exposed to high heats. Because of this, it's recommended that you use canola or olive oil, which are monosaturated fats, for cooking.

**6. Dairy (Dairy products can be categorized as fats, proteins, or carbohydrates.)**

*Maximum daily target: 8 ounces (1 cup)*

Like meat, dairy products come in saturated fat and unsaturated fat varieties. Again, the choice to use full fat, low fat or no fat is yours. The same argument about saturated fats versus unsaturated fats applies. Keep in mind, however, that many low-fat dairy products are loaded with high fructose corn syrup and/or sugar, especially the ones that are made with fruit. *Always* read the label before making your dairy choices.

## Summary of Sugar-Free Solution™ eating guidelines

| Category of Food | Daily Budget | Occasional Budget |
|---|---|---|
| **Grains** | 2 ounces | |
| **Fruits** | 8 ounces (1 cup) | Another 8 ounces (1 cup) occasionally |
| **Vegetables** | 32 ounces of nonstarch veggies | (includes up to 16 ounces of starchy vegetables per week) |
| **Poultry/Fish/ Meat/Eggs/ Hard Cheese/ Nuts/Seeds** | 12–16 ounces (depending on your weight target & gender) | |
| **Oils/Spreads** | As needed for cooking and flavoring | |
| **Dairy** | 8 ounces (1 cup) | |
| **Total Budget** | About 4 pounds of food every day | |

### Is it a healthy program?

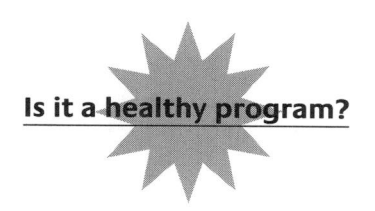

Let's figure this out by looking at the people who live to be one hundred years or older. This population category is called "centenarians," and a group of researchers at the Harvard Medical School are studying this population group to figure out what they did or did not do to make it to this age milestone. Other than being the recipients of "good" long-living genes, here are some common characteristics: Rather than aging more, centenarians are more successful at avoiding debilitating disease and injuries, particularly cardiovascular disease. Almost all centenarians have been lean for their entire lives, some naturally and some intentionally. Most of them never made a conscious effort to eat "nutritiously." Some drank alcohol, but many more didn't. Most never smoked. Most never saw a doctor until they were in their nineties. Several had never taken any medications whatsoever.

> The grim truth is that if you're overweight or if your weight constantly fluctuates, you have twice the risk of dying sooner than people with normalized weight.

Zoom in on the lifetime leanness characteristic, because that's what we're all after here. Lean means that your weight is proportional to your height. A lifetime of leanness means your body weight doesn't fluctuate. It stays the same—no ups and downs. Other than "good" genes, many researchers consider body weight to be the single most important predictor of longevity here on planet Earth. The grim truth is that if you're overweight or if your weight constantly fluctuates, you are a candidate for cardiovascular disease, hypertension, diabetes, and other weight-related conditions, which puts you at twice the risk of dying sooner than people with a normalized weight.

Individuals with weight problems are also the ones who are most likely to have injuries and other serious chronic diseases that compromise the quality and enjoyment of life such as problems with the back and joints, gout, osteoarthritis, constipation, and sleep apneas as well as depression and low self-esteem. From a long-term life perspective, normalizing and stabilizing your weight is one of the most important actions you can take to ensure that you stick around for a while. The Sugar-Free Solution™ will normalize and stabilize your weight.

But, you may ask, is the program a nutritionally sound one? At the turn of the last century, "good" nutritional advice was characterized by a focus on solving the problems of underconsuming or eating enough to meet basic, minimal needs. This has now completely reversed to a focus on solving the problems related to overconsuming. While there are many conflicting and ambiguous opinions about what constitutes "good" nutrition, there is consensual agreement that we should eat less and be more selective about what we choose to eat. The Sugar-Free Solution™ asks you to fulfill these objectives by providing you with "just right" portions *of all food types* as well as by cutting out all the excess that comes in the form of caloric sweeteners and highly processed foods.

The bottom line is that you do the best that you can for yourself with the limited and conflicting information that's available. One of the most useful tools you have available is your own mind. You can think for yourself. You can try different approaches and methodologies. And you can make your own decisions about what constitutes healthy eating.

## SECTION 2: GET SET

The whole point of The Sugar-Free Solution™ is to convince you that getting caloric sweeteners and other white stuff out of your diet is the single most important eating strategy you can make for yourself. But why take my word for it when you have the opportunity to prove it to yourself instead?

Do a short test and eliminate caloric sweeteners (plus white flour and white rice) from your diet for the next four weeks or twenty-eight days. Go about it in a somewhat scientific way by measuring your own "before and after" results. Start now by taking five baseline measures BEFORE you make any changes to your diet:

1. Your body weight

2. The size of the clothes you wear

3. Your waist measurement

4. Your blood chemistry
   - HDL Cholesterol
   - LDL Cholesterol
   - Triglycerides

5. Your own subjective feeling of health and well-being. Use a scale of 1 to 10 to rate your feelings, with one being the lowest and 10 being the highest.

Then live sugar-free for one full month and see for yourself how it feels and what happens. After the one-month period, retake the same measures. The goal of the experiment is to give you tangible, conclusive results that demonstrate how powerfully and quickly The Sugar-Free Solution™ works to shed pounds, lose inches, eliminate cravings, and improve your blood chemistry. Then you don't have to rely on promises from me or anyone else. And you don't have to guess which theory is right for you, because you will know.

## Comparison to USDA 2005 Revised Food Pyramid

For your convenience, a comparison of The Sugar-Free Solution™ food guidelines and the newly revised Food Pyramid, 2005 Dietary Guidelines for American adults, is provided below. It's published by U.S. Department of Agriculture. USDA amounts are presented in a range format, because different amounts of food are recommended depending on age and gender. For more detailed information, go to www.MyPyramid.gov.

| Type of Food | USDA Food Pyramid | Sugar-Free Solution™ |
|---|---|---|
| **Grains** | 5–8 ounces per day | 2 ounces per day |
| **Fruit** | 1½–2 cups per day | 1 cup per day (2 cups occasionally) |
| **Vegetables** | 2½–3 cups per day | 4 cups per day |
| **Dairy** | 3 cups per day | 1 cup per day |
| **Meat/Beans/Nuts/Seeds** | 5–6½ ounces per day | 12 to 16 ounces per day* |
| **Oils** | 5–7 teaspoons per day | (Oils/Spreads) As needed for flavor and cooking |
| **Discretionary** | 130–360 calories per day | No foods made with sugar or refined flours |

*Varies from 12 to 16 ounces, depending on your gender and target weight goal.

So, as you can see, The Sugar-Free Solution™ guidelines provide for more vegetables, more protein, and more oils/fat, but you will have less fruit, less grain, and less dairy. A basic premise of the USDA Dietary Guidelines is that nutritional needs should be met primarily by eating real foods rather than vitamins and supplements. This is also the basic premise of The Sugar-Free Solution™. Both programs make it possible to feed yourself with foods that are commonly found in grocery stores or farmstands.

## Your scale weight

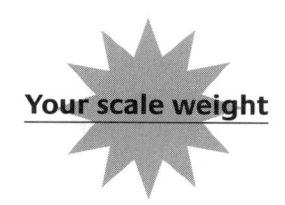

The Sugar-Free Solution™ is a way of eating that enables you to free yourself from the tyranny of food. Consequently, there's no reason to rush or to be anxious about your scale weight, because, in truth, you scale weight doesn't matter. What matters is how you eat, and that's where your attention should be. You will feed yourself this way before you reach your target scale weight. You will feed yourself this way when you reach your target scale weight. And you will feed yourself this way after you reach your target scale weight. So you see, your scale weight is irrelevant.

Make a decision now to put your scale weight on the back burner. Refuse to be driven by it. Refuse to weigh yourself more often than once a month. Refuse to talk about how much you weigh and/or how much weight you've lost or gained. Refuse to give your body weight a center stage position in your life. Instead, concentrate on how you feed yourself and how you feel about the way that you feed yourself. This sounds like a simple thing to do, but it's a monumental change in focus.

Your scale weight is an arbitrary number that symbolizes success to you. Yes, it's important and useful to have a goal. But now is the time to consider a different definition of success. How about if success is defined by your ability to eat within the food guidelines one "good" day at a time? If you follow the guidelines for one full day, you are successful. If you follow them another day, you are successful—and on and on. This makes it much faster and easier to experience success. All you have to do is live one "good" day. All the pressure to perform and to be a certain size drops away. This instantly makes the program doable, even enjoyable!

The other hidden advantage of living one "good" day at a time is that the goal never ends. Once you hit your scale weight, you won't go crazy and start eating anything and everything, just because you have achieved your goal, and now you're done with it. Instead, you're still locked into the goal of living a good day. The goal is still active. It's still directing you and keeping you calm and on track. Can you see how powerful and useful this change in focus can be to you?

# Questions and answers

**1. What happens if you eat something with sugar or white flour in it?**

What happens, if anything, depends on several factors: how much of it you eat, whether you're eating it as part of a meal or as a stand-alone snack, and the proportion of the sugar or white flour to the other substances in your meal. The most important question to answer is whether or not the sugar/white flour is a relatively minor, insignificant ingredient, or whether it's a dominant, primary ingredient.

If sugar is eaten as part of a meal, in a low dose where the sugar is not tasted in a strong way, you will probably not feel an effect from it.

If sugar is eaten as part of a meal, in a dose that's strong enough to taste, such as in a salad dressing or on an Easter ham, you may experience feelings of hunger or food cravings shortly after eating.

If sugar is eaten as a stand-alone snack or in a large dose such as a piece of cake or a candy bar, where the taste of sugar is obvious and dominant, you will most likely experience food cravings and hunger shortly after eating. You also may find yourself wanting more foods with sugar and find it hard to resist them. You may binge.

2. **Does this mean I can never have lasagna or spaghetti or pizza ever again?**

There are lots of choices available to you in the realm of pizza and doughs. One option for pizza or for calzones is to scrape the toppings off the dough and just eat the toppings. Another option is to make the dough yourself with a whole-grain or alternative type flour such as soy. And another option is to allow yourself to eat pizza rarely on special occasions.

Likewise, there are also several options for eating pastas. One is to substitute any green veggie for pasta and serve the sauce over it. This is absolutely delicious, and you will not miss the pasta! Another option is to buy or make whole-grain type pastas, but remember to limit the serving size to two ounces, which is much smaller than the full bowl of pasta you are used to. Or, the third choice, again, is to allow yourself to eat pasta foods, but only rarely on special occasions.

3. **How do I handle eating out at a restaurant?**

Eating out is easy. All restaurants in the U.S. offer protein and veggie choices, which makes it possible for you to find something to eat that's both satisfying and within the food guidelines. Pass on the bread or tortilla chips that come before the meal. Pass on food choices that involve pasta, breading, or stuffing. Ask for a double order of veggies, instead of the starch that is typically offered. Request a vinaigrette-type dressing on your salad. Avoid the low-fat or fat-free salad dressings, because there's a 99 percent chance they will be made with sugar or HFCS. Eat half of the protein if the portion being served to you is huge. It sounds complicated, but it's the same way you feed yourself when you're at home or anywhere else. Just relax into it.

4. **What about protein bars or low-carb bars?**

These snack foods are fine in a pinch. They're a better choice than allowing yourself to go hungry or grabbing something with processed flower and caloric sweeteners. Be sure to check the ingredients to make sure they're not made with sugar or HFCS. While you're at it, look at the long list of ingredients that don't seem to resemble food. Keep in mind that these bar-type foods are highly processed, and as we have discovered, processed foods don't usually turn out to be good for us.

**5. But what should I do if I'm on a limited budget? Eating in a sugar-free way is more expensive, and it's hard for me to allocate extra money for food.**

Yes, it's a little more expensive to eat fresh, high quality foods, but you are so worth the extra 10 or 15 percent cost. Also, if you take the time to shop sales, go to a food warehouse, and/or buy in bulk, the incremental cost of food can be minimized or even completely eliminated. You are not spending any extra money on meetings or expensive programs. It's all going directly to you and for you. Consider it an act of love for yourself. In any case, cost of food is no excuse. If you truly want to lose weight and to eat in a saner, healthier way, you will figure out a way to make it work.

**6. I don't just cook for myself; I also have to cook for my family. What if my family refuses to eat this way?**

Don't go to war over food. Explain what you are doing and why you are doing it, but do not force your eating style on anyone. Allow your family to watch you and see what happens. Your own demonstration of what works will be more powerful than any words you can speak and more persuasive than a useless argument.

## Decisions you make on your own

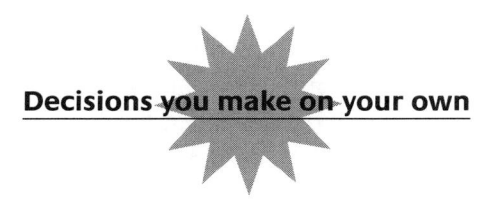

In addition to choosing whether to eat fat in a saturated or unsaturated form, there are other individual food decisions that you make all on your own. These decisions will be based on your own personal preferences and on your current beliefs about what constitutes a healthy eating lifestyle.

Here are your choices:

1. **Vitamins, minerals, supplements.** These substances have no impact on binge eating or weight. You decide whether or not to use them. If you elect to use them, just make sure to read labels and avoid anything that's made with sugar or sugar-like products. Also, be wary if the product has a calorie value. Many health practitioners think of taking vitamins as a kind of insurance that ensures daily mineral and vitamin requirements get met.

2. **Artificial substitutes for sugar.** There is constant controversy about the potential harm or harmlessness of eating sugar substitutes. What we do know is that, in the long run, man-made processed foods have turned out to be more of a health problem than a health problem solver. That said, it will be difficult to be successful on this program without some reliance on sugar substitutes. Currently, the only sugar substitute that you can

cook with is Splenda; products such as Equal or Sweet N Low break down when heat is applied. The choice of how much and how often to use these substances is up to you. However, it is advisable to reduce your reliance as much as practical and possible. That means try not to drink lots of diet soda when alternatives are available. Try not to eat foods that contain sugar substitutes at every single meal or snack. Try to reduce the amount of sugar substitute called for in recipes; usually, anywhere from one-fourth to one-half of the recommended amount can be left out with little difference in taste.

3. **Artificial substitutes for fats.** Naturally occurring fats are allowed on this program, so there's no need to choose these man-made products unless your doctor or healthcare practitioner has specifically asked you to do so. Of course, you can make the substitute if you want to, but why sacrifice the flavor and satisfaction if you don't have to? Also, once again, be wary of man-made substances.

4. **Alcohol.** Alcohol metabolizes as a carbohydrate and will definitely influence your insulin production. Even more importantly, alcohol makes it possible for you to forget your intention to eat in a sugar-free way. It's hard enough to hold a decision without the influence of alcohol. Some out-of-control eaters may also be out-of-control drinkers. One drink may lead to many. If you have difficulty limiting your alcohol intake, consider abstaining. In any case, if you choose to drink, limit your servings to one drink per day. Drink only at meals and never on an empty stomach. Do not consume beer, after-dinner liqueurs, or anything made with a mix that contains sugar.

SECTION 2: GET SET

5. **Fresh veggies versus frozen veggies versus canned veggies.** You make the choice for freshness or for availability and convenience.

6. **Caffeine.** Should you drink caffeinated coffee, decaffeinated coffee, or none at all? The most recent research suggests that up to three cups of coffee a day is okay for most people. In *Eat, Drink and Be Healthy*, author Walter C. Willet, MD, says, "In moderation . . . coffee is low on the totem pole of health risks." Of course, some people are more sensitive to caffeine than others. Beware, however, that most of the low-carb gurus believe that drinks made with caffeine can lead to an increase in insulin production.

7. **Salt.** The use of salt is yet another hotly debated topic. Our government and the American Heart Association recommend limiting salt intake to around 2,300 milligrams per day. The American Medical Association recently recommended further reducing this amount to 1,500 milligrams per day. As a reference point, just one teaspoon is about 1,900 milligrams of salt. A reduction in salt intake is particularly targeted at people who suffer from high blood pressure, which is currently defined as 140/90. However, many sport nutritionists recommend much higher amounts of salt intake for serious athletes, and researchers at the Albert Einstein College of Medicine say that *healthy people* who restrict salt to less than 2,300 milligrams per day are 37 percent more likely to die of cardiovascular disease. If you have high blood pressure or if you received salt intake advice from your healthcare practitioner, please follow the recommended guidelines. Otherwise, this is another one of those decisions that you make for yourself.

# SECTION 3: GO

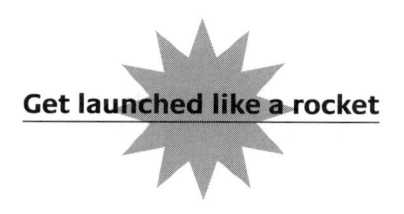

### Get launched like a rocket

There are only two things you need to do to get yourself started:

1. Make a decision.
2. Plan ahead.

**Make a decision and hold it**

Power comes from knowing exactly what you want. This is also known as "making up your mind" or "intending" to have or to do something. Your starting place is always to know, without any hesitation or doubt, your very own heart's desire. What is it you want, dear reader? Can you say it in words? Can you see it in your mind? Once you make a firm, unwavering decision about what you want, you are on your way to having it. Every decision produces a result of some kind. This is why it's an act of power.

Your decision literally and figuratively takes you where you want to go. You have already been successfully guided by your decisions many times in your life. You want a new car, and you get it. You want a new love interest, and one appears. It's the universal law of manifestation, and there's nothing mysterious or woo-woo about it. Everything comes to you through your decisions. The decision/intention functions like a strategic guide, which leads you toward some actions and away from others.

No special skills or abilities are required to make a decision and to intend something into manifestation. Everyone is able to do it. In fact, everyone intuitively already knows how to do it. The only hard part is holding your desire long enough to make it come about. We lose faith because we don't see the result right away. Or we see something that temporarily looks better. Or we forget. And just like that, in the very nanosecond that your mind changes, the result likewise changes. Let's say that you make a decision to abstain from sugar for a day. Then around 4 p.m. you make another decision to have a big bowl of ice cream made with high fructose corn syrup. The decision you made at 4 p.m. brings you a different result than the one you originally intended.

There are two little tricks for learning how to hold a decision:

1. Don't scare yourself by asking something that is still perceived as too much, too hard, or too long.

2. Acquire strength, confidence, and a pattern of success by holding your decision for short, easily doable but progressively longer and longer periods. So, for example, the first "holding" period that you ask of yourself might be a day or a week. The second "holding" period might be two weeks or a month. The third "holding" period might be two months or a quarter of a year or even a full year if you feel inspired. See how it works? Just ask yourself to take one small, doable step at a time.

Okay, let's get to it. The time is now to make yourself happy. No one else is going to do it for you. No one else CAN do it for you. There's no more procrastinating. No more dillydallying. No more wondering if you can or can't have what you want. Of course, you can. **Make the decision now** to abstain from any caloric sweeteners and from white flour and white rice for one full week. Start today or tomorrow or on the next Monday or on whatever day makes the most sense for you, but start.

SECTION 3: GO

*Say this phrase to yourself:* I will abstain from caloric sweeteners, white flour, and white rice for one full week, starting on _____ and ending on \_\_\_\_\_.

**Plan ahead**

It usually takes about forty-five minutes to get my nails done, but only about five or ten minutes is actually spent on painting them. The rest of the time is all allocated to prep work. If I wanted to skip the prep work and quickly jump to the part where I get my nails painted, they wouldn't look good. Even if the technician did the most perfect, painstaking painting job, the manicure would most likely still be marginal.

You also have some prep work to do. It will take more time for you to figure out what you're going to eat, how you're going to eat, and to prepare your food than it will take you to actually eat it. That said, you don't have to plan ahead a lot—one day ahead is fine, a few days ahead is even better, a week is ideal. But in any case, the time you spend planning will make it easier and more enjoyable for you to eat foods that you love and to preempt eating mistakes.

The first thing you need to do is to buy a food scale. It doesn't have to be an expensive, fancy brand. It just has to be a scale that you can easily read. This eating program is based on eating a "just right" volume of food, which is measured in ounces. Therefore, it's essential that you become familiar with what an ounce of meat looks like, or what an ounce of nuts looks like, or what an ounce of sugar-free brownie looks like. You'll be tempted to skip this step and to "wing" the quantities, but don't. Remember, you're on a remedial training program. You're relearning how to feed yourself. One of the things you need to relearn is what a "just right" quantity looks like. Eventually, you'll be able to approximate measures based on what you see, but for now it's best to measure, measure, measure. That way you won't be either underfeeding yourself or overfeeding yourself.

The next thing you need to do is clean out your refrigerator and your pantry. Check the ingredients list of all those low-fat products in your refrigerator. Weed out the ones that are made with high fructose corn syrup and sugar. Get rid of all the highly processed, sugar-based foods that might tempt you: cookies, cakes, candy, chips, and the like. If you have a habit of drinking calorically sweetened drinks, get rid of them, too. Throw the food out, give it away, or feed it to the birds. Just get it out of your space. A time will come when it doesn't matter whether or not these foods are present, but, for now, at the start of the program, it will be easier for you to get them out of sight and out of reach.

Then figure out what you're going to eat for the first five days on the program. Use the menus in the book as a starting point, but fine-tune these to your tastes and preferences. If you absolutely hate planning and cooking, then make it as easy as possible for yourself.

Buy frozen, chopped veggies rather than dealing with fresh ones. Consider having the same breakfast, the same lunch, and the same snacks for a week at a time. That way, all you have to really plan for is dinner. This practice of eating the same thing several days in a row will go against the grain of every nutritionist. They will tell you that it's healthier to eat a variety of foods, but sometimes it's more important to be just plain practical rather than worrying about nutritional correctness. Your end task is to make up a shopping list based on what you plan to eat. Use *Go Tool #5: Start-up Shopping List* as a starting point, but tinker with it. Make it yours.

After you go shopping, prepare some foods ahead of time. Take an evening or a weekend afternoon and get yourself ready. Clean and chop up lettuces and store them in a zip-locked bag. Grill or roast a batch of several days' worth of veggies. Make one or two salad dressings for the week. Measure out nut quantities and put them in little baggies or containers. Make your sugar-free brownies and the baked zucchini snack.

## Now get going

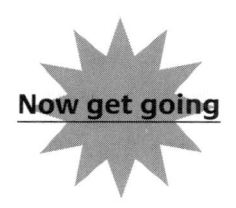

You've got everything you need to be successful. You've got the latest and greatest information. You've got the go tools. You've already made a firm decision to abstain for a pre-determined period of time. There's nothing holding you back. Quit waiting around for happiness to come to you. Instead, start living in a way that will make you happy. Happiness is experienced in the very moment you stop attacking yourself with food and start feeding yourself in a loving way.

Nothing is impossible, dear reader. Your body will respond to your request for change. It willingly accommodated your request to store fat, and it will likewise willingly accommodate your request to shed it. Ask it kindly. Treat it kindly. Never give up.

I look forward to receiving your personal success story.

## GO TOOL #1: Meal planning tips

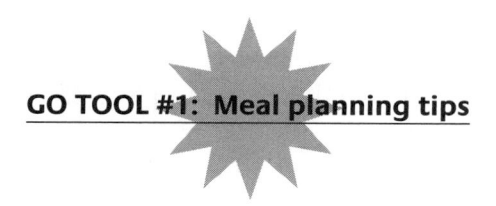

Meal planning is one of those activities that's relished if you love to cook and hang out at the grocery store, and dreaded if you don't. These planning guidelines are especially intended for all the busy people who don't have a lot of time to devote to meal planning, shopping, or cooking and might be tempted to skip over the planning process. The secret is to do planning tasks that generate batches of food that will serve you for at least several days or possibly for a whole week.

For example, instead of eating a different breakfast every single day, and thus planning seven different breakfasts and shopping for seven different breakfasts, have the same breakfast from Monday through Saturday. That way, you only have to think about two different breakfasts: your Sunday breakfast and your Monday–Saturday breakfast. Plan your lunches in a similar way. Except, as a variation, you might want to consider giving yourself three lunch choices instead of two. You have your Monday–Wednesday–Friday lunch, your Tuesday–Thursday–Saturday lunch, and your Sunday lunch (or your lunch that you eat out). Likewise, cook a dessert and/or prepare snacks and salad ingredients that you can eat for several days in a row. Then you only have to deal with one daily, variable meal that must be planned, and that's dinner. This takes all the stress out of having to come up with twenty-one different meals and twenty-one different snacks each week.

Lunches and dinners will usually include a protein, a vegetable, and a salad of some kind, and that gets pretty easy to plan around. So your biggest meal planning decisions are when to have your daily grain, daily dairy, and daily fruit budget. Some people like to have grain (cereal) and dairy (milk) in the morning for breakfast and then have a piece of fruit for a mid-morning snack. Other people, like me, prefer to have grain as a mid-afternoon snack (in the form of a delicious chocolate brownie or something else that's equally yummy) and dairy and fruit as an evening "to die for" homemade ice cream dessert. There's no better or worse way to do it. All you have to do is figure out what makes sense for you, your lifestyle, and your personal preferences.

The examples that are provided here show two different plans. They're both based on a daily protein budget of 14 ounces. The first one is for a day that starts out with grain and dairy in the morning, and the second one is for a day that ends with dairy and fruit in the evening. Many other combinations are also possible. For example, you might occasionally want to have a cream-based soup as part of your dinner for your dairy budget; you might prefer a dairy-based smoothie for a snack in the afternoon; or you might like to have your grain as a dessert in the form of a couple scrumptious homemade sugar-free cookies.

Try to keep in mind that the guidelines are just that: guidelines. It may not always be possible to eat the types of foods in the exact recommended volume amounts. Use the guideline as a general target and do the best you can.

SECTION 3: GO

## EXAMPLE #1

| Meal | Amount and Type Food |
|---|---|
| Breakfast | 2 oz. grain (such as whole grain cereal)<br>6 oz. dairy (such as low-fat milk) |
| Mid-morning snack | None |
| Lunch | 6 oz. protein<br>4 oz. cooked veggies<br>8 oz. salad |
| Snack | 2 oz. protein<br>4 oz. veggies |
| Dinner | 6 oz. protein (with 2 oz. cream sauce)<br>8 oz. cooked veggies<br>8 oz. salad |
| Dessert | 8 oz. fruit |

## EXAMPLE #2

| Meal | Amount and Type Food |
|---|---|
| Breakfast | 2 oz. protein (omelet)<br>4 oz. veggie |
| Mid-morning snack | Grain with spread |
| Lunch | 6 oz. protein<br>4 oz. veggies<br>8 oz. salad |
| Afternoon snack | 2 oz. protein<br>4 oz. veggies |
| Dinner | 6 oz. protein<br>8 oz. cooked veggies<br>8 oz. salad |
| Dessert | 6 oz. dairy (homemade ice cream)<br>8 oz. fruit |

THE SUGAR-FREE SOLUTION™

**Weekly planning and preparation tasks**

*Planning Decisions*

1. Your Monday–Saturday breakfast

2. Your Monday–Wednesday–Friday lunch
   Your Tuesday–Thursday–Saturday lunch

3. Your snack(s) for the week

4. Your dessert(s) for the week

5. Your six of seven dinners that you will cook for the week. *These choices are just examples. Choose dinners based on your own preferences.*
   - ❑ 1 chicken
   - ❑ 1 beef
   - ❑ 1 fish
   - ❑ 1 pork
   - ❑ 1 ethnic
   - ❑ 1 super-fast and easy

*Preparation Tasks*

1. Clean, cut, and bag greens for salads.

2. Make or buy two different sugar-free salad dressings.

3. Roast or grill enough vegetables or buy enough microwaveable vegetables for four or five days.

4. Make or buy your grain and snacks for the week.

5. Pre-measure out snacks, and put them in little bags or containers so that you won't be tempted to overeat.

# SECTION 3: GO

**The first month is the most time-consuming month**

It will take you a while to read food labels, to find new sugar-free products that you love, and to try out recipes that work for you and your family. After about a month, magic happens. Planning, shopping, and food prep all get easier. Give yourself the gift of time to learn this new, life-changing eating system.

## GO TOOL #2: Sample daily menus

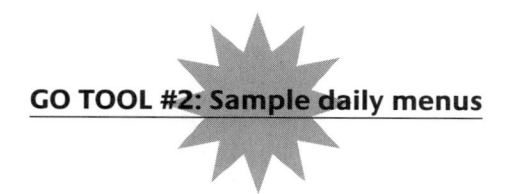

Here are three simple examples that show how a daily menu can be put together. They are all based on a fourteen-ounce budget of protein per day. Ingredients feature familiar foods that most people like. There is nothing "sacred" about these menus. They are provided for two reasons: 1) to give you an idea of how to go about the meal planning process, and 2) to let you know how I "count" food types. As you will see, I count by predominant food type and try not to get too hung up on figuring out the exact values for small portions of ingredients that are used in recipes. The total daily food volume is always within two or three ounces of the target, one way the other. Beverages are not listed. Drink water or any nonalcoholic beverages that have not been calorically sweetened.

If you must drink alcohol, limit it to one drink of wine or hard spirits, at your main meal.

## MENU #1

| | |
|---|---|
| *Breakfast* | Western omelet with salsa<br>*2 oz. protein*<br>*4 oz. cooked veggies* |
| *Mid-morning Snack* | 1 piece baked zucchini snack<br>*2 oz. grain* |
| *Lunch* | Cucumber, tomato, red onion salad<br>*8 oz. raw veggies* |
| | Green beans flavored with bacon<br>*4 oz. cooked veggies* |
| | Chicken satay<br>*4 oz. protein* |
| *Mid-afternoon snack* | Spiced nut mix<br>*2 oz. protein* |
| *Dinner* | Mesclun salad mixed with roasted peppers and artichokes<br>*8 oz. raw veggies* |
| | Sautéed scrod with tartar sauce<br>*6 oz. protein* |
| | Sautéed Brussels sprouts<br>*4 oz. cooked veggies* |
| *Dessert* | Homemade mixed berry "ice" cream<br>*8 oz. fruit*<br>*4 oz. dairy* |
| **TOTAL** | 56 ounces of food<br>3.5 pounds |

## MENU #2

*Breakfast*

Fried egg
*1 oz. protein*

Mushrooms sautéed with thyme
*4 oz. cooked veggies*

*Mid-morning snack*

Plain yogurt mixed with fresh peach
*6 oz. dairy*
*8 oz. fruit*

*Lunch*

Tuna salad
*4 oz. protein*

Grilled or roasted veggie medley
*4 oz. cooked veggies*

Salad of romaine, radicchio and Parmesan shavings
*8 oz. raw veggies*
*1 oz. protein*

*Mid-afternoon snack*

Cheese and pepperoni
*2 oz. protein*

*Dinner*

Hearts of palm and mesclun salad
*8 oz. raw veggies*

Bolognese sauce over sautéed asparagus
*6 oz. protein*
*8 oz. cooked veggies*

*Dessert*

Sugar-free brownie
*2 oz. grain*

---

**TOTAL**

62 ounces of food
3.8 pounds

## MENU #3

| | |
|---|---|
| *Breakfast* | Broccoli, bacon & cheese quichette<br>*4 oz. protein*<br>*2 oz. cooked veggies* |
| *Mid-morning snack* | A medium-sized piece of fruit (other than a banana)<br>*8 oz. fruit* |
| *Lunch* | Deli meat roll-ups<br>*4 oz. protein*<br><br>Grilled or roasted veggie medley<br>*4 oz. cooked veggies*<br><br>Homemade coleslaw<br>*8 oz. raw veggie* |
| *Mid-afternoon snack* | Baked zucchini snack with cream cheese<br>*2 oz. grain* |
| *Dinner* | Spinach salad with sun-dried tomatoes and feta cheese<br>*8 oz. raw veggies*<br>*1 oz. protein*<br><br>Chicken with prosciutto, artichokes and asparagus<br>*5 oz. protein*<br>*4 oz. cooked veggies* |
| *Dessert* | Sugar-free cheesecake<br>*6 oz. dairy* |
| **TOTAL** | 56 ounces of food<br>3.5 pounds |

## GO TOOL #3: Recipes

**BREAKFAST**

**Western Omelet with Salsa**

*Ingredients: (serves 1)*

    1 egg
    1 ounce of your favorite cheese, grated
    1 ounce each of green peppers, red pepper, and onions, finely chopped
    Olive oil
    1 tablespoon of water
    Salt and pepper to taste
    Your favorite brand of sugar-free salsa

*Directions:*

In a bowl, mix egg with water. Add salt and pepper. Mix.

In a nonstick frying pan, add 1 tablespoon of oil and veggies, sauté for 2 or 3 minutes until soft. Add egg mixture. Shake frying pan. Lift edges to allow uncooked egg to cook.

When top is almost firm, sprinkle on cheese.

Fold in half. Cook one more minute. Slide onto plate and serve with salsa.

## Broccoli, Bacon and Cheese Quichettes

*Ingredients:*

- 1 cup of frozen broccoli flourettes
- 3 strips cooked, crumbled bacon
- 3 eggs
- 6 ounces of shredded cheese (cheddar, Monterey jack, or your favorite)
- 2–3 scallions, finely chopped
- 1 cup heavy cream
- Salt and pepper to taste
- 5 drops Tabasco (optional)

*Directions:*

Preheat oven to 350 degrees. Line the muffin pan with foil baking cups and spray them with oil Microwave the flourettes for 2½ minutes on high. Drain excess liquid. Cook bacon in microwave for 3 minutes. Dry on paper towel and crumble.

In a bowl, combine the eggs and cream and mix. Then add cheese, broccoli, and bacon. Add salt, pepper, and Tabasco if desired. Mix well. Divide evenly among muffin cups. Bake for 20 minutes or until a knife inserted in center comes out clean. Serve hot, warm, or room temperature. May be frozen and reheated in microwave (remove foil)

## SNACKS

### Baked Zucchini Snack
*Using George Stella's excellent technique for cooking with soy flour.*

*Ingredients:*

> Vegetable oil cooking spray
> 3 cups shredded zucchini with skin on
> ½ cup onions, finely chopped
> 2 tablespoons parsley, chopped
> 1 clove garlic, crushed
> ½ cup olive oil
> ½ cup Parmesan cheese, grated
> ½ teaspoon pepper
> ½ teaspoon salt
> 1 teaspoon oregano
> 4 large eggs, beaten
> 1½ cup soy flour (plus 2 tablespoons soy flour)
> ¼ cup wheat bran
> ½ cup club soda
> 1½ teaspoon baking soda

*Directions:*

Preheat oven at 375 degrees. Spray a 9 x 13 x 2 baking dish. Mix the wheat bran and 2 tablespoons of soy flour together. Evenly coat baking dish with this mixture. In a bowl, blend all the remaining ingredients. Pour into the baking dish. Bake at 375 for 25–30 minutes or until knife inserted into the center comes out clean. Freezes well. Serve plain or with cream cheese.

## VEGGIES

*You're going to be eating a lot of veggies, so it's worth taking the time to prepare them in ways that are flavorful and delicious*

### Sautéed Mushrooms
*Great at breakfast or as a side vegetable at lunch or dinner.*

*Ingredients:*

- 1 8-ounce package of any kind of fresh mushrooms or mushroom mixture
- 2 tablespoons of olive oil
- ½ teaspoon of thyme
- Salt and pepper

*Directions:*

Heat the oil in a small frying pan. Add the mushrooms to oil and sprinkle with thyme. Sauté over high heat until golden brown, turning every minute, cooking for a total of about 5 minutes.

Add salt and pepper and serve.

### Grilled or Roasted Veggie Medley
*Cook a large batch ahead and make enough for several meals.*

*Ingredients:*

- (any combination of vegetables you prefer)
- Spanish onions, sliced in thick rounds
- Eggplant, sliced in long strips
- Green and red peppers, sliced in thick strips
- Zucchini, sliced in long strips
- Asparagus spears
- Olive oil
- Salt and pepper to taste

*Directions:*

Prepare veggies and coat with oil. Sprinkle with salt and pepper.

For grilling: Put on a hot grill. Turn once after a couple of minutes.

For roasting: Put on a cookie sheet. Roast in 450-degree oven for 15–20 minutes, no turning is necessary.

## Sautéed Brussels Sprouts

*Even people who hate Brussels sprouts, love these.*

*Ingredients:*

>1 pound Brussels sprouts, cleaned with "X" cut in bottom
>2 tablespoons olive oil
>3 tablespoons good balsamic vinegar
>1 tablespoon Parmesan cheese, grated
>Salt and pepper to taste

*Directions:*

In a pot, boil the Brussels sprouts for 8 minutes. Remove from water. Cut in half. Set aside. Put oil in a large frying pan and heat.

Put Brussels sprouts in pan cut-side down. Sauté for 2 or 3 minutes.

Add balsamic vinegar, salt, and pepper. Sauté 2 or 3 minutes longer. Add cheese and serve.

## SALAD AND SALAD DRESSING

### Homemade Coleslaw

*Ingredients:*

>2 cups green cabbage, shredded
>2 cups red cabbage, shredded
>1 carrot, shredded
>¼ red onion, finely chopped
>2–3 scallions, thinly sliced

*Dressing:*

>½ cup mayonnaise
>½ cup sour cream
>1 tablespoon apple cider vinegar
>1 teaspoon Splenda
>1 or 2 drops of Tabasco (optional)
>Salt and pepper

## Balsamic Parmesan Dressing

*Makes enough for several servings.*

*Ingredients:*

⅓ cup best balsamic vinegar you can afford
⅔ cup extra virgin olive oil
2 cloves garlic, crushed
1 tablespoon Parmesan cheese, grated
1 teaspoon spicy brown mustard
½ shallot, finely chopped
1 teaspoon salt
½ teaspoon freshly ground black pepper

*Directions:*

Mix in a food processor or blender until oil is emulsified.

*Variation:*

Add 2–3 tablespoons of coursely chopped sun-dried tomatoes after the dressing is emulsified.

SECTION 3: GO

## DINNERS

### Bolognese Sauce

*This recipe is a little complicated, but so worth it. It will satisfy your cravings for pizza and pasta, and your family will love it. This batch is large enough for several meals. It freezes well. Measure out your sauce portion and then serve it over your favorite veggie, which has been cooked in any way that you prefer or that's most convenient for you (steamed, sautéed, grilled).*

*Ingredients for sauce:*

- 2 tablespoons olive oil
- 6 strips of bacon, diced
- ½ pound ground sausage
- 1 pound ground beef
- 1½ cups onions, chopped
- ½ cup carrots, finely chopped
- ½ cup celery, finely chopped
- ¼ pound mushrooms, thinly sliced
- 3 cloves garlic, minced
- 1 cup Chablis
- 3 cups chicken stock
- 1 teaspoon salt
- ¼ teaspoon black pepper, freshly ground
- ½ cup heavy cream
- ¼ cup fresh parsley, chopped

*Directions:*

Heat olive oil in large frying pan over medium heat. Add onions, carrots, celery, and mushrooms. Cook and stir often for about 5 minutes, until soft. Add garlic, cloves, nutmeg, and cook for another 1 or 2 minutes. Remove from heat and set aside. In a large pot, cook bacon over high heat until light brown. Add ground meats and cook, stirring constantly, until browned. Add vegetable mixture and tomato paste and cook for 2 minutes. Add Chablis and cook until almost evaporated. Add chicken stock and simmer over medium-high heat until sauce is thick and flavorful (about 45 minutes to 1 hour). Add salt and black pepper. Stir in cream and parsley.

## Chicken with Prosciutto, Artichokes, and Asparagus

*Ingredients:*

- 4 boneless, skinless chicken breasts, pounded to ¼-inch flat
- ¼ cup unsalted butter
- 2 tablespoons olive oil
- 1 can (14 ounces) artichoke hearts, packed in water, drained and halved
- 4 slices prosciutto, medium thickness
- ¼ cup Parmesan cheese, freshly grated (Regianno recommended)
- 1 cup chicken stock (canned is okay)
- 2 tablespoons parsley, chopped
- 16 fresh asparagus, cooked al dente
- Salt and pepper to taste

*Directions:*

Put chickens in between two pieces of wax paper and pound flat to approximately ¼-inch thick. Season with salt and pepper. Heat butter and oil in a large frying pan and sauté the chicken for about 10 minutes, turning once, until they are a golden color. Sprinkle chicken with the ½ of the Parmesan cheese. Lay one piece of prosciutto on each piece of chicken. Sprinkle with remaining Parmesan cheese and parsley. Add chicken stock and artichokes. Cover and cook for 8 to 10 minutes. Boil or steam the asparagus while chicken is cooking. Arrange pieces of chicken on dinner plate. Pour pan juice over top and garnish with 4 asparagus spears on each piece.

## DESSERTS

### Mixed Berry "Ice" Cream
*This is so incredibly good. You will never even slightly miss ice cream made with sugar and trans fats.*

*Ingredients:*

    1 cup frozen mixed berries
    1 cup crushed ice (small cubes are also okay)
    ½ cup heavy cream
    ⅛ cup Splenda
    1 teaspoon sugar-free vanilla extract

*Directions:*

Put all the ingredients into a food processor. Manually do about 60 short pulses. Then switch to high and blend another 60 seconds until ice chunks are smoothed. Makes 2 servings.

## GO TOOL #4: Food selection guidelines

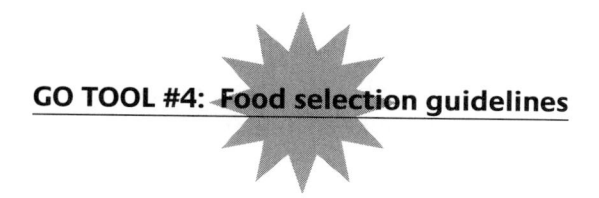

Food selection guidelines are based on the carbohydrate value and/or the glycemic index of foods. It's not necessary, however, to count carbohydrates or to study the glycemic index of everything you put in your mouth. All you need is a general understanding of the science behind the food selection process and some guidelines regarding the three types of food categories:

- Category #1: Low carbohydrate and very low glycemic index foods

- Category #2: Mid-range carbohydrate and glycemic index foods

- Category #3: High carbohydrate and glycemic index foods

### Carbohydrates

The carbohydrate category includes all foods that have natural sugar in them, which cuts across all vegetables, all fruits, all grains and bakery products, and some dairy. The lower the carbohydrate gram count, the less the natural sugar in the food.

### Glycemic index

The glycemix index, which is also referred as the GI, is a system for measuring how fast a carbohydrate triggers an immediate rise in your blood glucose level. Carbohydrates that have a high GI likewise have a high, fast impact on glucose. Carbohydrates that have a low GI have a slow, low impact on blood glucose.

The concept of a glycemic index was introduced about twenty-five years ago and is still a relatively new and emerging field. Glucose is arbitrarily assigned a value of 100, and all other foods are measured relative to that value. Some foods have a range of values because of differences in growing and/or cooking procedures. For example, an apple grown in France might have a different GI than an apple grown in the U.S. The University of Sydney provides a free, online searchable database of foods that have been tested by the university's researchers for a GI value. If you want to know more about the GI in general, or if you'd like to track down the value of a specific food, go to www.glycemicindex.com.

**Category #1: Low carbohydrate and very low glycemic index foods**
*GI of less than 25*

- **Proteins:** There are no GI values for meat, poultry, fish, cheese, or eggs because they contain so little carbohydrates that they're not likely to induce a significant increase in glucose.

- **Fats:** There are no carbohydrates in fats or GI values for fats.

- **Most vegetables grown above the ground (except corn):** Above-the-ground veggies with very low GI indexes include artichokes, asparagus, Brussel sprouts, cabbages of all kinds, cauliflower, cucumbers, celery, eggplant, green beans, lettuces and "greens" of all kinds, mushrooms of all kinds, peppers of all kinds, snow peas, summer squash, tomatoes, zucchini.

- **Most nuts and seeds (except cashews).**

As you already know, proteins and vegetables are your primary source of nutrition on The Sugar-Free Solution™ program. You will be eating approximately three pounds of food each day from these low carbohydrate and very low GI sources. This is roughly 75 percent of your total daily food intake.

**Category #2: Mid-range carbohydrates and glycemic index foods**

*GI of greater than 25 and less than 70*

- **Most fruits (except bananas, pineapple, and watermelon):** includes apples, apricots, berries of all kinds, cantaloupe, cherries, grapefruit, honeydew melon, lemons/limes, orange, papaya, peach, pear, plum, strawberries.

- **Most dairy products.**

- **Most root vegetables** except potatoes (baked, fried, or boiled), parsnips, and rutabaga, which all have a GI greater than 70.

- **High fiber whole grain cereals, pastas, and baked products** that are made without caloric sweeteners (or very little of them).

You can enjoy grains, fruits, dairy, and root vegetables on a regular basis on The Sugar-Free Solution™ program, but these are foods that you must be more careful with. They collectively account for approximately one pound or 25 percent of your total daily intake.

**Category #3: High carbohydrates and high glycemic index foods**

*GI of greater than 70*

- **Dates, bananas, pineapples, mango, watermelon.**

- **Potatoes, parsnips, rutabaga, corn, pumpkin.**

- **Most snack foods and processed foods** including popcorn, chips, cookies, cereals and bakery products.
- **Most candies.**
- **Calorically sweetened drinks.**

The Sugar-Free Solution™ program makes it possible for you to enjoy high carbohydrate/high GI fruits and vegetables once in a while, on special occasions. However, highly processed baked products, candies, and calorically sweetened drinks are not allowed.

# GO TOOL #5: Start-up shopping list

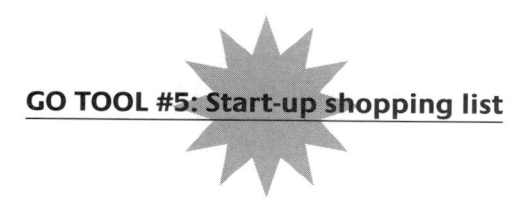

**PROTEIN CHOICES**

*Note: If low saturated fats are important to you, choose lean versions of meat and low-fat versions of cheeses.*

| Type of Food | Frequent Choice | Occasional Choice |
|---|---|---|
| **MEATS** | Beef | |
| | Chicken | |
| | Turkey | |
| | Capon, Cornish Hen | |
| | Pork | |
| | Ham (but not baked or cured with sugar) | |
| | Bacon | |
| | Veal | |
| | Lamb | |
| | Sausage | |
| | Hotdogs | |
| | Lunch Meats (not cured with sugar) | |
| | | |
| **FISH AND SHELLFISH** | Fish—all kinds | |
| | Shellfish—all kinds | |

# THE SUGAR-FREE SOLUTION™

| Type of Food | Frequent Choice | Occasional Choice |
|---|---|---|
| **EGGS** | Whole Eggs (not limited unless directed by your healthcare practitioner) | |
| **CHEESES** | Hard Cheeses including American, Cheddar, Monterey, Mozzarella, Muenster, Parmesan, Provolone, Swiss, String | |
| | Ricotta | |
| | Feta | |
| | Cottage Cheese | |
| **NUTS** | Almonds | |
| | Brazil Nuts | |
| | | Cashews |
| | Hazelnuts | |
| | Macadamia | |
| | | Peanuts |
| | Pecans | |
| | Pine Nuts | |
| | Pistachios | |
| | Walnuts | |
| **SEEDS** | Sesame | |
| | | Pumpkin/Squash |
| | | Sunflower |

SECTION 3: GO

*Note: If low saturated fats are important to you, choose non-fat or low-fat versions of dairy products. But be sure to check the ingredients list of these lower fat products for the presence of caloric sweeteners.*

| Type of Food | Frequent Choice | Occasional Choice |
|---|---|---|
| **DAIRY** (In general, there are fewer carbohydrates in dairy products with a higher fat content. The decision to include or avoid fat is up to you.) | Skim or Low-fat Milk (1% or 2% fat) = 11.7 carbohydrates per cup | |
| | Whole Milk (3.7% fat) = 11.4 carbohydrates per cup | |
| | Buttermilk = 11.7 carbohydrates per cup | |
| | Soybean Milk = 5.8 carbohydrates per cup | |
| | Plain Whole Milk Yogurt = 10.6 carbohydrates per cup | |
| | Half & Half = 9.6 carbohydrates per cup | |
| | Light Cream = 9.6 carbohydrates per cup | |
| | Heavy Cream = 8.0 carbohydrates per cup | |
| | Sour Cream = 8.0 carbohydrates per cup | |
| **OILS & SPREADS** | Olive Oil | |
| | Canola Oil | |
| | Cooking Spray Oil | |
| | Butter | |
| | Mayonnaise | |
| | Cream Cheese | |

## THE SUGAR-FREE SOLUTION™

| Type of Food | Frequent Choice | Occasional Choice |
|---|---|---|
| **GRAINS** | White Flour alternatives such as soy flour or almond flour | |
| | Multi-grain Breads (3 grams of fiber and sugar is 4th ingredient or more on list) | |
| | Rice, brown or wild | |
| | Whole Grain Cereals, made without sugar | |
| | Whole Wheat Pasta | |
| | Whole Wheat or Stone Ground Pita | |
| | | Whole Grain Bagels, small or half |

## SECTION 3: GO

| Type of Food | Frequent Choice | Occasional Choice |
|---|---|---|
| **FRUITS** | Apple | |
| | Apricot | |
| | | Bananna |
| | Berries—all kinds | |
| | Canteloupe | |
| | Cherries | |
| | | Dates |
| | | Grapes |
| | Grapefruit | |
| | Honeydew Melon | Kiwi |
| | Lemons/Limes | Mango |
| | Orange | |
| | Papaya | |
| | Peach | |
| | Pear | |
| | Plum | |
| | | Pineapple |
| | Strawberries | |
| | | Watermelon |

# THE SUGAR-FREE SOLUTION™

| Type of Food | Frequent Choice | Occasional Choice |
|---|---|---|
| **VEGGIES** | Asparagus | |
| | Artichokes | |
| | Avocado | |
| | Beets | |
| | Bok Choy | |
| | Broccoli<br>Broccoli Rabe<br>Broccolini | |
| | Brussel Sprouts | |
| | Cabbage—<br>all kinds | |
| | | Carrots |
| | Cauliflower | |
| | Celery | |
| | Collard Greens | |
| | | Corn |
| | Cucumbers | |
| | Eggplant | |
| | Fennel | |
| | Garlic | |
| | Green Beans— all kinds | |
| | Green Peas | |
| | Lettuce—<br>all kinds | |
| | Mushrooms— all kinds (even dried) | |
| | Olives—<br>all kinds | |
| | Onions, Scallions, Leeks—<br>all kinds | |
| | | Parsnips |

## SECTION 3: GO

| Type of Food | Frequent Choice | Occasional Choice |
|---|---|---|
| | Peppers—all kinds | |
| | | Potatoes |
| | Radishes | Pumpkin |
| | | Rutabaga |
| | Snow Peas | |
| | Spinach | |
| | Sprouts | |
| | Squashes—all kinds | |
| | | Sweet Potatoes |
| | | Yams |
| | Tomatoes (fresh and sugar-free canned) | |
| | | Turnips |
| | Water Chestnuts | |
| | Zucchini | |

# THE SUGAR-FREE SOLUTION™

| Type of Food | Frequent Choice | Occasional Choice |
|---|---|---|
| **OTHER** | Food Scale | |
| | Paul Prudhomme's Meat Magic | |
| | Sugar-free Vanilla Extract | |
| | Sugar-free Salsa | |
| | Baking Powder & Baking Soda | |
| | Mustards: brown, Dijon, yellow, whole grain | |
| | Vinegars: balsamic, red wine, sherry | |
| | Spices including basil, oregano, thyme, sage, nutmeg, chili powder, salt, pepper | |
| | Capers | |
| | Chicken & Beef Broth | |
| | Splenda | |
| | Tomato Paste | |
| | Fresh Herbs such as basil, parsley, rosemary | |

# GO TOOL #6: Recommended products, cookbooks and reading list

## PRODUCTS

**Soy Flour**

It's worth every minute of your time to shop around for a great soy flour such as Bob's Red Mill Organic Whole Grain Soy Flour, which can be found in most health food stores and occasionally at grocery stores. Unlike other similar flours, Bob's doesn't have a strong soy smell or flavor, and it's also very moist. As it turns out, these are two critically important qualities when you're making the switch from white flour to soy flour. The other soy flour brands that I've tried have not been as tasty, and the foods that I made with them sometimes have a dry and crumbly texture. Get Bob's. You'll love it.

**Balsamic Vinegar**

Buy the best aged balsamic vinegar that you can afford. My favorite is Rao's Home Made Balsamic Vinegar from Modena, Italy. It's been aged twelve years and is very pricey, but the flavor and consistency is superior to other lower-priced, less-aged brands.

**Olive Oil**

So long as you're going to eat fat, make it really good fat. Colavita Extra Virgin Olive Oil is one of the most delicious olive oils commonly available in the grocery store. My husband and I buy several liters at a time and use it for salad dressings and every type of cooking. The flavor is wonderful and will definitely make a difference in the way the foods that you cook taste. Again, it's a little pricier than other oils, but worth the cost.

**Meat Seasoning**

My husband is a talented cook, and he's always reminding me that good food is all about good seasoning. Paul Prudomme's Meat Magic is one of those amazing products that makes all kinds of meats taste really delicious, no matter how skilled or unskilled you are at cooking. Meat Magic has no sugar, additives, preservatives, or MSG. It can be found in some grocery stores and also at http://shop.chefpaul.com.

**Noncaloric Sweeteners**

The only noncaloric sweetener product that you can cook with is Splenda. The standard measures for sugar and Splenda are exactly the same. One tablespoon of sugar is equivalent to one tablespoon of Splenda. This makes Splenda easy to use and easy to adapt in your favorite recipes. However, be aware that Splenda is very sweet, and because of that, the quantities recommended for most recipes can be cut by one-fourth to one-half without any taste difference.

**Sugar-free Vanilla**

It's difficult to find vanilla brands that aren't made with sugar. The best ones are made with both sugar and bourbon, which dramatically enhances the flavor. Spice Islands has both qualities: great flavor and no sugar! Frontier Vanilla Extract is usually available in any health food store and can sometimes be found in the health food section of your grocery store.

**Canned Tomato Products**

Note that food manufacturers are inconsistent about the use

of sugar in their canned tomato products. Some products are made without caloric sweeteners, and others aren't. Your best bet is always to check the ingredients label. Here are the brands that I use:

Hunts Whole Tomatoes
Tuttoroso New World Style Crushed Tomatoes
Pastene Ground Peeled Tomatoes Chunky Style

**Noncaloric Drinks**

I should buy stock in Polar Seltzer water, because I drink several liters of its "bubbly water" every day. Polar Seltzer comes in many different flavors, and they're all good. I'm particularly fond of Mandarin Orange. Be aware that Polar makes different types of carbonated waters products, so be sure to look for the ones that say "no calories" on the front label. If you're in doubt, again, check the ingredients label on the back to make sure that you're selecting one that does not include any caloric sweeteners.

## COOKBOOKS

Use your favorite cookbooks for meat/chicken/fish dishes, soups, veggies, and salads. Simply substitute Splenda for any sweetener (including honey) and pass on recipes that call for pasta, white flour, and white rice. The best place to look for recipes for pasta alternatives, desserts, baking products, and sugar-free sauces is in the low-carb section of your favorite bookstore or at www.amazon.com.

Keep in mind, however, that your goal is not low-carb eating, but rather to simply eliminate caloric sweeteners, white flour, and white rice from your diet. Also, be aware that terms like "low-carb" and "carb-smart" and "net carbs" don't have standard definitions, and, therefore, cannot be relied on. You will find so-called low-carb recipes that list sugar and/or white flour and sweetened chocolate as ingredients. Disregard these recipes and look for something else. You also will find low-carb cookbooks that include ingredients such as Atkins mix, protein whey mix, sugar-free pudding mixes (which are full of trans fats), crushed low-carb food bars and other sometimes hard-to-find substances. None of these products are necessary, but some people prefer them. It's up to you to decide whether or not you want to use these types of foods.

### George Stella's Livin' Low Carb: Family Recipes Stella Style

If you can only afford to buy one cookbook, this is the one to get. Stella's recipes are so unusually good because he and his wife are both professional chefs, and they know how to put foods together in a no-fail, delicious way. Stella uses soy flour for his baking products rather than prepared mixes, which I personally prefer. I've tried about twenty recipes from this cookbook, and every single one of them is great.

### Cookbooks by Suzanne Somers

Somers is the queen of sugar-free cooking. The author of six fine cookbooks, she has a talent for combining ingredients in unexpected, fresh ways. Foods are made with ingredients that can easily be found in any grocery store. Ignore the food combining recommendations and "level" distinctions and go straight to the food section. You can use Splenda instead of SomerSweet. Here are Somers' cookbooks:

- *Suzanne Somers' Fast & Easy*
- *Suzanne Somers' Get Skinny on Fabulous Food*
- *Suzanne Somers' Eat Great, Lose Weight*
- *Suzanne Somers' Eat, Cheat and Melt the Fat Away*
- *Suzanne Somers' Slim & Sexy Forever*
- *Somersize Desserts: 30 Fantastic Recipes for Sumptuous, Great-tasting, Guilt-free Treats*

SECTION 3: GO

### Low Carb Energy Magazine

This publication is a great resource for new recipes and up-to-date information about sugar-free foods. It's available four times a year, although sometimes is it difficult to find at newsstands or in grocery stores. For more information, visit www.lowcarbmagazines.com.

### Carb Lite Magazine

This is another excellent resource for interesting recipes and articles. Published six times a year, it is also hard to find. For more information, visit www.carblitemag.com.

## READING LIST

### The Diet Wars

*Featured on Frontline by PBS (www.pbs.org/wgbh/pages/frontline/shows/diet/)*
This program focuses on "the fattening of America." It asks why it's happening and what can be done. A wide range of experts, from various backgrounds, is interviewed. The end result is a big picture perspective that doesn't favor any one solution.

### Eat Fat, Lose Weight: How the Right Fats Can Make You Thin for Life

*By Ann Louise Gittleman, ND, CNS, with Dina R. Nunziato, CSW*
Gittleman presents a strong case for eating all naturally occurring fats and for avoiding all trans fats. She goes into detail about Omega fats and oils. Published by Keats Publishing, 1999.

### Lick the Sugar Habit

*By Nancy Appleton, PhD*
Appleton says that disease is our leading growth industry in the U.S. and that sugar is the cause of it. Her book is the most frequently quoted source about the metabolic dangers of sugar. Published by Avery Publishing Group, 1996.

**Protein Power**

*By Michael R. Eades, MD, and Mary Dan Eades, MD*

If you want more science, this book gives it to you—in spades. The Eades are two physicians who specialize in weight loss. This explains their approach and also gives the reader extensive background research information about why low-fat diets fail and how they lead to obesity and other health problems. Published by Bantam, 1996.

**Eat, Drink and Be Healthy: The Harvard Medical School Guide to Healthy Eating**

*By Walter C. Willett, MD, co-developed with The Harvard School of Public Health*

Willett and company give the reader a consolidation of the latest research and findings related to diet and health. While Willett does not embrace a full sugar-free approach for weight loss and weight management, he is at least open to the possibility that insulin plays a role and that fat is not always the villain. Published by Free Press, 2005.

# GO TOOL #7: Common FDA food terms

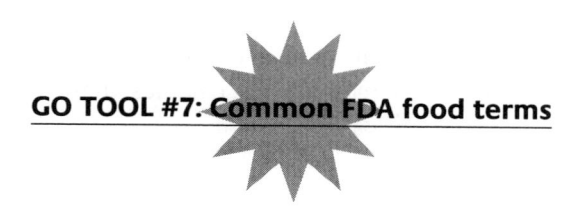

The Food and Drug Administration has standardized certain food-related terms and now mandates that food manufacturers meet the defined criteria before the terms can be used in packaging. The terms are listed here for your convenience and handy reference. As you will see, it is a well-intended but thoroughly confusing effort, and it's unlikely you will remember most of the terms. This situation is further compounded by the fact that several undefined food terms are also used, and food manufacturers have the freedom to use these terms in any way they want to use them. The undefined terms are also included in this reference list.

There is no need to rely on any of these labels. Instead, get into the habit of reading the ingredient listing that must appear on any packaged or processed food and make your own assessment about whether or not the food is appropriate for you.

**Free, Zero, No**
Means that a product has none of the substance.

**Insignificant, Negligible**
Means that a product has so little of a substance that it's hardly measurable.

**Low**
Means that this food could be eaten often without exceeding daily limits for calories, fat, saturated fat, cholesterol, and/or

sodium. This is also sometimes expressed as "little" or "low source of."

**Reduced**
Means that the food contains at least 25 percent of the featured macronutrient or 25 percent fewer calories than the regular product.

**Light, Lite**
Means that the food contains either one-half the fat or sodium or one-third the calories of the regular product.

**High**
Means that the product has 20 percent or more of the nutrient or vitamin than minimum daily value. This is also sometimes expressed as "rich in" or "excellent source of."

**More**
Means that the food has 10 percent more of the minimum daily nutrient or vitamin than the original product.

**Good Source**
Means that the food has somewhere between 10 to 19 percent of the daily requirement for a nutrient or vitamin.

**Fruit**
The term "fruit" could be used for any of the following substances: real fruit, fruit juice, fruit concentrate, fruit syrup, high fructose corn syrup (HFCS).

**Whole Grain**
Not defined. Check the ingredients listing to make sure that the first ingredient is a whole-wheat flour rather than a plain wheat flour, unbleached wheat flour, or enriched wheat flour. Also check the fiber count. A truly "whole" product will have at least 3 grams of fiber per serving.

### Low-carb
No standardized definition.

### Net carb
No standardized definition.

### Glycemic index
No standardized definition.

### Serving size
No standardized definition. Beware that many manufacturers "undersize" their listed portions, which then distorts the posted nutritional information. Again, your best bet is always to read the ingredient listing and to measure your own portions.

### Pure
No standardized definition.

### Healthy
No standardized definition.

### General claims about improvements to health
No requirements for food manufacturers to substantiate these claims through the FDA.

### Qualified claims about improvements to health
Must be backed by preliminary or emerging scientific evidence. Currently "qualified" health claims are limited to omega-3 fatty acids found in fish, nuts, and olive oil.

## SECTION 4: STAY IN TOUCH

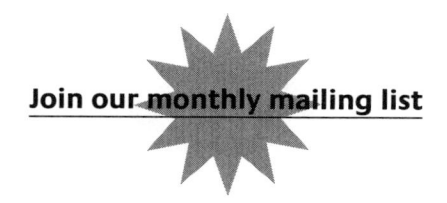

**Join our monthly mailing list**

Be a part of our growing family of active program participants by subscribing to our mailing list. Just send your name and e-mail address to expert@getextremeresults.com. This information will not be rented, shared, or sold, and that's a promise! And you will not be bombarded with constant e-mails either. If you change your mind later on, it's super-easy to unsubscribe. All you have to do is ask.

Everyone who subscribes receives a free report, *The 10 Biggest Mistakes to Avoid When Trying to Lose Weight.* Then, once a month you get a content-rich newsletter filled with:

- A sugar-free success story
- A new sugar-free recipe
- A recent Q&A about living the sugar-free program
- A tip and inspiration for staying on track
- The GETEXTREMERESULTS boot camp and seminar schedule
- Any new or special product offerings that you might want to know about

The e-newsletter is a convenient and easy way to stay motivated and for us to keep in touch. Go to your computer and sign up now.

## Send your endorsement or tell your story

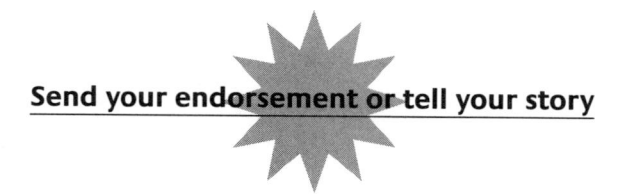

If, after reading this book, you feel inspired to write an endorsement or to share your personal success story, I welcome it. Your comments and/or story will be posted at the www.GETEXTREMERESULTS.com web site.

Please contact the expert@getextremeresults.com to find out more about the special treats and rewards that are offered to endorsers and to those who share their stories.

You can send your information in any way that is convenient for you:

**By e-mail: expert@getextremeresults.com**

**By fax: 603.253.4801**

**By U.S. mail: P.O. Box 1209, Center Harbor, NH 03226**

It will be my great pleasure to read about your personal experience.

Until then, remember that I am rooting for you.

## Come to a GETEXTREMERESULTS Boot Camp

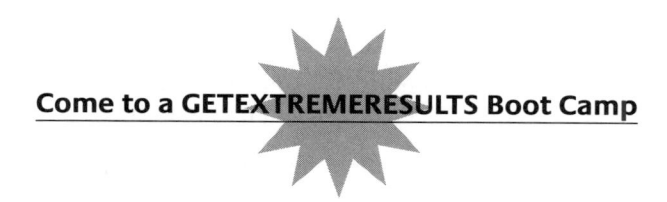

*When:* Boot camps are usually scheduled once a month, except for July, August, and December when the program is not offered.

*Where:* Check www.GETEXTREMERESULTS.com for locations.

*How Long*: Each boot camp runs a full day from 9:30 a.m. to 4:30 p.m. and includes a delicious, satisfying sugar-free lunch, snacks, and beverages.

*Here's what you get:*

- All the information contained in this book and lots more
- The opportunity to fully define your new self
- A chance to meet and be inspired by Karen Bentley
- New *Sugar-Free Solution*™ recipes
- A live cooking demonstration of sugar-free foods, especially desserts, snacks, and alternative grain foods (which you will be able to sample)
- All your personal questions about the sugar-free program answered

*You also will be able to:*

- Develop your own customized start-up meal plan
- Learn how to create weekly and monthly shopping lists
- Learn how to select and/or modify recipes from your favorite cookbooks to make them sugar-free
- Learn how to make sugar-free choices from any menu in a restaurant
- Learn how to recover from mistakes and keep yourself on track no matter what
- Get energized with an easy exercise routine that can be adapted for home use
- Laugh, have fun, and connect with others on the same path

Please bring a notepad and pen or pencil. Also please wear loose, comfortable clothing that is suitable for mild exercise.

## Share your favorite sugar-free recipes

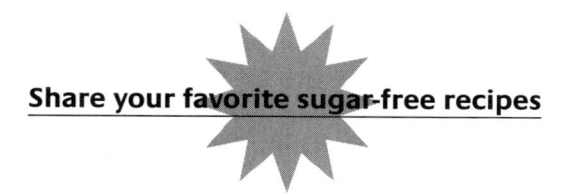

The best part about The Sugar-Free Solution™ is that you can eat delicious foods. If you're one of those creative people who gets pleasure from experimenting in the kitchen and coming up with new recipes, please consider sharing them with The Sugar-Free Solution™ family of participants.

Anyone who sends an original recipe that's selected for publication on our web site or in an e-newsletter will be paid $25. Anyone who sends an original recipe that's selected for a printed publication will be paid $100. Recipes that are sent to us become the property of GETEXTREMERESULTS and will not be returned.

When submitting a recipe, please be sure to name it, to list all the ingredients, and to provide cooking or assembly directions. Also include your own name, phone, e-mail address, and U.S. mail address so that we can contact you to let you know if the recipe has been selected or if we have questions about it. E-photos of you and/or the food in .jpg format are welcome.

Send your recipes in any way that's convenient:

**By e-mail: expert@getextremeresults.com**

**By fax: 603.253.4801**

**By U.S. mail: P.O. Box 1209, Center Harbor, NH 03226**

## Acknowledgments

Any English 101 teacher will tell you that decent writing comes about through revising, revising, and more revising. For me, at least, it's unlikely that the first words I put down on paper will say exactly what I mean in a way that's easy and interesting for people to read. This is why it's so essential for me to work with others to produce a final product that comes out clear, well-organized, and polished.

I am grateful to my talented editor, Sherry Roberts, for refining my work, for ensuring that I adhere to a consistent style, and for suggesting a different and more powerful ending to the book.

I am grateful to my readers: Charlotte Brook-Signor and Donna Ulbright, two of the smartest women I know, for their interest in the project and for helping me to fill in the gaps with information that was missing or that originally was presented in a way that didn't grab or hold their attention.

And most of all, I am grateful to my husband, the fabulous Bill Bentley, for supporting me through the time-consuming writing process whether I was doing the writing at home, on a cruise, or on vacation and for helping me to develop delicious, tested recipes that anyone can follow.

One of the most enjoyable aspects of writing a book is that I get to express my appreciation to so many wonderful people. Love is the way I truly walk in gratitude.

XXOO
KB